QR コードで動画が見られる!

歯科医学英語ワークブック
第 2 版

Answers
（解答編）

JN097126

金芳堂

Lesson 1: Treatment Procedures

上村先生のワンポイントアドバイス

患者は治療中にストレスを受けています。これは疲労や不快感に繋がる可能性があり、歯科医はこのストレスを軽減するように努めなければならない。的確な指示は治療の流れを円滑にします。その結果、患者と歯科医師双方にとって良い治療になります。

1. Core Terms

1. open 2. close 3. bite down 4. open wide 5. keep open 6. relax 7. rinse out
8. 手順 9. 下げる 10. 上げる 11. バキューム 12. 治療

4. Core Phrases

1. チェアを倒します。
2. お口を開けてください。
3. お口を大きく開けてください。
4. お口を開けたままにしてください。
5. 噛み合わせてください。
6. お口を閉じていいですよ。
7. お口をゆすいでください。
8. チェアを戻します。

6. Risa's Coffee Break

Question: "What's this area?"
Answers: This is the <u>waiting room</u>. （こちらは待合室です）
          This is the <u>reception</u>. （こちらは受付です）
          This is the <u>treatment room</u>. （こちらは治療室です）
          This is the <u>operation room</u>. （こちらは手術室です）
          This is the <u>laboratory</u>. （こちらは技工室です）
          This is the <u>office</u>. （こちらは院長室です）

7. Workout

1. You have bad breath.
2. You have periodontitis.

8. Dialogs

Dialog 1

Dentist: もしもし。
Patient: Hello? I don't have an (appointment)...but can I see you (right) (away)?
         もしもし。予約していませんが、すぐに診ていただけますか。
Dentist: What seems to be the problem?
         どうなさいましたか。
Patient: I have a (terrible) (toothache).
         歯がひどく痛みます。
Dentist: Oh, no. Please come (right) (away). May I have your name?
         それはいけません。すぐに来てください。お名前は。
Patient: My name is Peter Parker.
         私の名前はピーター・パーカーです。
Dentist: OK, Mr. Parker, don't forget to bring your (insurance) (card).
         ではパーカーさん、保険証を忘れずに。
Patient: Sure. I will be there (in) (ten) minutes.
         わかりました。あと 10 分くらいで到着します。

Dialog 2

Dentist: How is the (weather) outside?
　　　　外の天気はどうですか。

Patient: It's a (beautiful) day though a bit (chilly).
　　　　きれいに晴れていますが少し肌寒いです。

Dentist: So, how did you get here?
　　　　どうやって来たのですか。

Patient: I walked from the train station.
　　　　駅から歩きました。

Dentist: Must have been (tough) finding your way.
　　　　見つけるのに苦労されたのでは。

Patient: Actually, it was a (breeze).
　　　　いや、すごく簡単でしたよ。

Dentist: You didn't ask anyone (on) (the) (way)?
　　　　途中で道を尋ねなかったのですか。

Patient: No need. My smartphone (app) guides me in English. See?
　　　　その必要はないです。スマホのアプリが英語で案内してくれます。ね？

Dentist: Wow!
　　　　すごい！

9. Listening Comprehension （巻末 Answer Sheet）

Dialog 1

Q 1. What is the patient problem?　患者は何で困っているのか。
　　　He has a terrible toothache. (He also does not have an appointment.)
　　　彼はひどい歯痛がある。（彼はまだ予約をしていない。）

Q2. What must he bring to the clinic?　彼は来院の時に何を持参する必要があるのか。
　　　He must bring his insurance card.
　　　彼は健康保険証を持参する必要がある。

Dialog 2

Q1. How is the weather?　どのような天気なのか。
　　　The weather is beautiful but a bit chilly.
　　　いい天気だが少し肌寒い。

Q2. How did the patient find his way to the clinic?　患者はどのようにして医院までたどり着いたか。
　　　He used his smartphone app.
　　　彼はスマホのアプリを使った。

10. Test （巻末 Answer Sheet）

1. open　2. close　3. bite down　4. open wide　5. keep open
6. rinse　7. procedure　8. lower　9. raise　10. treatment

Lesson 2: General Terms

上村先生のワンポイントアドバイス　学生時代に多くの歯科用語を学びました。しかし、患者を診始めると、多くの場合においてこれらの用語が通じないことに気付きました。患者に説明をする時は、"gingiva," "caries," "orthodontic device"（専門用語）ではなく "gums," "cavity," "braces"（一般用語）を使うようにしました。

1. Core Terms

1. treat 2. tooth / teeth 3. cavity 4. dental clinic 5. dentist 6. Dentistry 7. 脱落 8. 萌出
9. 乳歯 10. 永久歯 11. 着色

4. Core Phrases

1. A dental clinic is where you get your teeth treated.
   歯科医院は歯の治療をうける場所である。
2. The hygienist assisted the dentist during the checkup.
   歯科衛生士は検診の時に歯科医の補助をした。
3. This treatment requires several visits.
   この治療は数回の来院を必要とする。
4. The primary teeth start to erupt from about 6 months of age.
   乳歯は生後 6 か月から萌出する。
5. Baby teeth shed at various times during childhood.
   乳歯は幼年期中の様々な時期に脱落する。
6. Permanent teeth begin erupting at 6 years of age.
   永久歯は 6 歳頃から萌出し始める。
7. Dental students study Dentistry at dental school.
   歯学部生は、歯学部で歯科医学を学ぶ。

5. Quick Response

歯科医院 dental clinic　衛生士 hygienist　検診 check-up　来院 visit　乳歯（専門用語）primary teeth　萌出 erupt　生後 6 か月 six months of age　乳歯（一般用語）baby teeth　脱落 shed　永久歯 permanent teeth　歯学部生 dental (school) student　歯学 Dentistry　歯学部 dental school

6. Risa's Coffee Break

Question: What are these?　これは何ですか。
Answers: These are incisors.（切歯）→ These are canines.（犬歯）→
　　　　　 →　These are premolars.（小臼歯）→　These are molars.（臼歯）

7. Workout

1. (front) (teeth) = anterior teeth　前歯
2. tartar = (calculus)　歯石
3. cavity = (caries)　カリエス
4. (baby) (teeth) = primary teeth　乳歯
5. adult teeth = (permanent) (teeth)　永久歯
6. (gum, gums) = gingiva　歯肉
7. bite = (occlusion)　咬合
8. (back) (teeth) = posterior teeth　後方歯
9. braces = (orthodontic) (appliance)　矯正装置
10. (wisdom) (tooth) = third molar　第三大臼歯

8. Dialogs

Dialog 1

Peter:　Bill, when was the last time you had a (checkup) (at) the dentist?
　　　　ビル、最後に歯科検診を受けたのはいつだ？
Bill:　A few years back when I was in the United States. Why?

数年前、まだアメリカにいた時に。なぜ？

Peter: Well, I noticed you have (a) (lot) (of) (stains) on the front of your teeth.
前歯にステインがいっぱい付いているよ。

Bill: Yeah, I think I'm...maybe I am drinking too much (coffee) (and) (wine). Is it that bad?
ああ、コーヒーやワインの飲みすぎかな。そんなに付いている？

Peter: It's pretty bad recently. Why don't you (visit) my (dentist)? He is very skilled and the (hygienist) does a wonderful job.
最近、目立つね。僕の歯医者さんはどう？上手だし、衛生士さんもいい仕事をするよ。

Bill: Can they speak English?
英語は通じるの？

Peter: They can.
通じるよ。

Bill: Really? Okay, great. So, tell me where are they?
本当？それはいいね。どこにあるの？

Peter: Here, I can show you.
これで教えてあげるよ。

Dialog 2

Bill: Have you been to a (dental) (clinic) in Japan?
日本で歯科医院へ行ったことはある？

Peter: Yes, I visit (one) (twice) (a) (year).
あるよ。年に2回行くよ。

Bill: Is the dentist skilled and easy to (communicate) (with)?
歯科医の腕は？話しやすい？

Peter: Yes, and he speaks English well.
うん、しかも英語が上手だ。

Bill: Sounds nice. That means you can ask about (treatment), (options), and (procedures)?
それはよさそうだ。ということは治療や選択肢や内容について聞けるのか？

Peter: Yes, that's why I am a (regular) (patient).
そう。だからいつも利用しているんだ。

9. Listening Comprehension（巻末 Answer Sheet）

Dialog 1

Q1. What did the friend notice about his teeth?　歯を見て友人は何に気づいたのか。
He has a lot of stains on his front teeth.　前歯にステインがいっぱいついている。

Q2. What seems to be the cause of the problem?　（ステインの）原因は何か。
He is drinking too much coffee and wine.　彼はコーヒーとワインを飲み過ぎている。

Q3. What does the man like about his dentist?
彼はいつも利用している歯科医の何が気に入っているのか。
He is very skilled and speaks English.（歯科医は）とても上手で英語も話せる。

Dialog 2

Q1. How often does he visit a dental clinic?　彼はどれくらいの頻度で歯科医院を訪れるのか。
He visits twice a year.　彼は年に2回訪れている。

Q2. What does this man like about his dentist?　彼は歯科医のどこが気に入っているのか。
He is skilled and easy to communicate with.　彼は上手で話しやすいから。

10. Test（巻末 Answer Sheet）

1. tooth (teeth) 2. cavity 3. dental clinic 4. dentist 5. Dentistry
6. shed 7. erupt 8. primary teeth (baby teeth) 9. permanent teeth (adult teeth) 10. stains

Lesson 3: Parts of the Mouth

上村先生のワンポイントアドバイス　学生時代は英語単語を見て覚えました。つまり、単語カードの表に英単語、裏面に日本語訳を書きました。英単語を見て、瞬時に和訳を言うようにしました。実際には、外国人患者は英語を話すときに単語カードを見せてくれません。だからヒアリング力を上げることは重要です。

1. Core Terms

1. tongue   2. lip(s)   3. cheek(s)   4. upper jaw   5. lower jaw   6. 粘膜   7. (顎) 関節
8. 歯肉   9. 歯根   10. 歯冠   11. 犬歯   12. 臼歯   13. 小臼歯   14. 切歯   15. 唾液

4. Core Phrases

1. 犬歯で食べ物を引きちぎる。   2. 臼歯で咀嚼中に食べ物をすりつぶす。
3. 切歯で食べ物を小さく切る。   4. 小臼歯で食べ物をちぎってつぶす。
5. 歯肉は歯の根元を覆う組織である。   6. 歯は歯冠と歯根に分けることができる。

6. Risa's Coffee Break

ホッチキス - stapler　→　ピンセット - tweezers　→　マーガリン - margarine　→　レンジ - microwave oven　→　チャック - zipper　→　→　リュックサック - backpack　→　マンション - apartment　→　キシリトール - xylitol　→　タバコ - cigarette　→　オランダ - Netherlands

7. Workout

1. 味わう、食べる、話すなどの機能に使われる筋組織。tongue
2. 口の入り口を形成する 2 つのひだ。lips
3. 顔の両側にある柔らかな部分。cheeks
4. 歯の歯根を囲む組織。gums
5. 口を形作る 2 つの骨。jaws
6. 口の中に分泌される潤滑、咀嚼、嚥下のための液体。saliva

8. Dialogs

Dialog 1

Patient: Hello. May I talk to the dentist? (It's) (an) (emergency).
　　　　　もしもし。歯科医はいますか？緊急です。

Dentist: Hello. What happened?
　　　　　もしもし。どうなさいましたか。

Patient: I was eating a sticky pecan pie and my crown (came) (off).
　　　　　ペカンパイを食べていたらクラウンが外れました。

Dentist: Did you (swallow) it?
　　　　　飲み込んだのですか？

Patient: Fortunately not. I have it here in my hand.
　　　　　幸い飲み込んでいません。手に持っています。

Dentist: You must come to the clinic (right) (away).
　　　　　今すぐ医院へ来てください。

Patient: But I can't. I am on vacation. Is it o.k. if I (put) (it) (back) (on) with some adhesive like superglue?
　　　　　無理です。今休暇中で。瞬間接着剤のようなもので付け直しても大丈夫ですか？

Dentist: No! Don't do anything like that.
　　　　　だめです。そのようなことは絶対にしないでください。

Patient: Then I will see you when I return (the) (day) (after) (tomorrow). In the meantime what should I do?

では明後日、戻った時に行きます。それまでに何をすればよろしいでしょうか？

Dentist: (Be) (sure) (to) keep it clean by brushing softly. O.K.? Your tooth might be (sensitive) (to) hot or cold drinks and food.

そっと磨いて清潔に保ってください。歯が熱いものや冷たいものに敏感かもしれません。

Patient: Gotcha. Thanks, doc.

了解です。ありがとう、先生。

Dialog 2

Dentist: Hello, Peter.

ピーターさん、こんにちは。

Patient: Hello, Doctor. You are going to treat my cavity today, right?

先生、こんにちは。今日は虫歯の治療でしたよね。

Dentist: That's correct. (Anything) (wrong)?

そうですよ。何かありましたか。

Patient: Well, something hurts on the inside of my (left) (cheek).

実は、左頬の内側が痛いです。

Dentist: Let's take a look...Oh, you have a large (canker) (sore).

診ましょう。大きな口内炎がありますね。

Patient: It hurts pretty bad. Can we (postpone) treatment?

かなり痛いです。今日の治療を延期できますか。

Dentist: Yes. I think that's a good idea. I will (disinfect) the sore and (prescribe) some steroids.

はい。その方がいいと思います。口内炎を消毒してステロイドを処方しておきます。

Patient: OK.

はい。

［注］pecan pie ＝ ペカンナッツとコーンシロップで作る甘いパイ

9. Listening Comprehension（巻末 Answer Sheet）

Dialog 1

Q1. What kind of emergency is it?　どのような緊急事態なのか。

His crown came off. クラウンが外れた。

Q2. What did the patient suggest?　患者は何を提案したか。

He suggested to put it back on with superglue. 接着剤で付けることを提案した。

Q3. Until treatment is available, what precautions should be taken by the patient?

（来院して）治療ができるまで、患者が気をつけるべき点は何か。

The patient should keep the site clean by brushing softly.

患者はそっと歯磨きをすることにより患部を清潔に保つ必要がある。

Dialog 2

Q1. Where is the canker sore?　口内炎はどこにできたのか。

It is on the inside of his left cheek. 左頬の内側にできた。

Q2. What will the dentist do?　歯科医はどのように対処するのか。

He will disinfect the sore and prescribe some steroids.

彼は口内炎を消毒してステロイドを処方する。

10. Test（巻末 Answer Sheet）

1. tongue 2. joint 3. gum(s) 4. roots   5. crown
6. canine 7. molar 8. premolar 9. incisor 10. saliva

Lesson 4: Interview

新人歯科医として一生懸命したことは、患者にとって「過剰」であることも。一方で、時間に追われた結果、「過少」になることも。どのような治療においても、正確さと一貫性が最も重要だと思います。

1. Core Terms

1. patient interview   2. hurt   3. ache   4. blood   5. bleed   6. 鈍い痛み
7. 鋭い痛み 8. ズキズキする痛み 9. ～に対して敏感   10. 麻痺した   11. 神経
12. ぐらつく感じがする   13. 違和感 14. 腫れた歯肉 15. 抜歯

4. Core Phrases

1. どうなさいましたか。
2. 当院は初めてですか。
3. どこが痛みますか。
4. いつから痛みますか。
5. どのような痛みですか。
6. 抜歯をしたことはありますか。
7. その時は何か問題は起きましたか。

6. Risa's Coffee Break

Question: What's this?

Answers: 1. This is enamel. これはエナメル質です。/ 2. This is dentin. これは象牙質です。/ 3. This is pulp. これは歯髄です。/ 4. This is the periodontal membrane. これは歯根膜です。/ 5. This is cementum. これはセメント質です。/ 6. This is the alveolar bone. これは歯槽骨です。/ 7. This is gingiva. これは歯肉です。

7. Workout

1. There are heavy stains on your front teeth.
2. There is a possibility of tooth decay.

8. Dialogs

Dialog 1

Dentist: What seems to be the problem?
どうなさいましたか。

Patient: My tooth aches especially when I eat (solid) (food).
特に固い食べ物を食べると歯が痛みます。

Dentist: Is this your first visit to this clinic?
当院は初めてですか。

Patient: Yes, it is.
はい、そうです。

Dentist: Where is the pain?
どの歯が痛みますか。

Patient: It seems to be in one of my (upper) (right) (teeth). I think it is the (second) (one) from the back.
右上の歯のうちどれかのようです。後ろから2番目の歯だと思います。

Dentist: When did the pain start?
いつから痛んでいますか。

Patient: About last week when I was (chewing) on some nuts.
先週、ナッツを食べた時からです。

Dialog 2

Dentist: What kind of pain is it?
どのような痛みですか。

Patient: It's a (slight) (pain) except when I chew on it. Then, it is a (sharp) (pain).
かすかな痛みです。しかし（その歯で）噛むと鋭い痛みです。

Dentist: Have you ever had a tooth extraction?
抜歯をしたことはありますか。

Patient: Extraction?
抜歯？

Dentist: Removed.
歯を抜くことです。

Patient: Yes, I had a (wisdom) (tooth) taken out.
はい。親知らずを抜いたことがあります。

Dentist: Did you experience any problems then?
その時何か問題は起きましたか。

Patient: No.
いいえ。

9. Practice 及び 10. Role Playing （巻末 Answer Sheet）

1. What seems to be the problem?　どうなさいましたか。
    Case 1 I have a toothache.　歯が痛みます。
    Case 2 I have a toothache.　歯が痛みます。
2. Is this your first visit to this clinic?　当医院は初めてですか。
    Case 1 Yes, it is.　はい、そうです。
    Case 2 Yes, it is.　はい、そうです。
3. Where is the pain?
    Case 1 It is in my lower left in the back.　左下の奥です。
    Case 2 It is in my upper right, the second from the back.　右上です。後ろから 2 番目の歯です。
4. When did the pain start?　いつから痛みますか。
    Case 1 It started last night.　昨晩から痛み出しました。
    Case 2 It started last week.　先週から痛み出しました。
5. What kind of pain is it?　どのような痛みですか。
    Case 1 It is a sharp pain.　鋭い痛みです。
    Case 2 It is a dull pain.　鈍い痛みです。
6. Have you ever had a tooth extraction?　抜歯をしたことはありますか。
    Case 1 Yes, I have.　はい、あります。
    Case 2 Yes, I have.　はい、あります。
7. Did you experience any problems then?　その時に、何か問題は起きましたか（経験しましたか）。
    Case 1 No, I didn't.　いいえ。（経験していません）
    Case 2 No, I didn't.　いいえ。（経験していません）

Lesson 5: Interview 2

上村先生のワンポイントアドバイス

患者の方のアレルギーがないことを確認することは特に重要なことです。時々アレルギーは思わぬトラブルを引き起こします。一部の薬に対するアレルギー反応は命を脅かしかねません。金属もアレルギーを引き起こします。

1. Core Terms
1. blood pressure   2. allergy   3. health insurance   4. 副作用   5. 投薬   6. 麻酔薬
7. 糖尿病   8. 妊娠中   9. 蓄積   10. 症状   11. 花粉症   12. 歯石

4. Core Phrases
1. 何かアレルギーはありますか。
2. 投薬により副作用を経験されたことはありますか。
3. 妊娠されていますか。
4. 他に気になることはございますか。
5. 保険証はお持ちですか。
6. 他にご希望や気になることはございますか。

6. Risa's Coffee Break
おはよう - Good morning   → こんばんは – Good evening   → こんにちは – Good afternoon   → 調子はどう – How are you doing?   → 今日はどうでしたか – How was it today?   → 今日はいい天気ですよね – Nice weather today.   → 風が強いですよね – The wind is strong, isn't it?

7. Workout
1. Q : What are you allergic to? あなたは何に対してアレルギーを持っていますか。
   A : I am allergic to eggs. / I am allergic to cats. / I am allergic to anesthetic.
2. Q : Do you have any allergies? アレルギーはありますか。
   A : I have food allergy. / I have hay fever. / I have metal allergy.
3. Q : What are your symptoms? 症状は何ですか。
   A : I have itchiness. / I have a fever. / I have a stomachache. / I have rashes.

8. Dialogs
Dialog 1
Dentist: Do you have any allergies?
          アレルギーはありますか。
Patient: I have (hay) (fever), otherwise no.
          花粉症以外はありません。
Dentist: Have you experienced any side effects from medication?
          投薬による副作用は経験されたことはありますか。
Patient: No, I haven't.
          ありません。
Dentist: Are you pregnant?
          妊娠されていますか。
Patient: Yes, I am (three) (months) (pregnant).
          はい。妊娠3か月です。

Dialog 2
Dentist: Is there anything else that bothers you?
          他に気になることはありますか

Patient: No, only this (toothache).
いいえ。この歯痛だけです。

Dentist: Do you prefer treatment for just this problem? Or, are there any other problems?
この治療だけをご希望されますか。それとも他にありますか。

Patient: It has been a while since I had my (tartar) (removed). Could you check for any (buildup)?
以前歯石をとってからしばらく経ちます。付いているか診ていただけますか。

Dentist: Do you have health insurance?
健康保険に入っていますか。

Patient: Yes, I am (insured).
はい、入っています。

9. Writing Practice 及び 10. Interview and Role Playing （巻末 Answer Sheet）

1. Do you have any allergies?　アレルギーはありますか。
    Case 1　I am allergic to eggs.　私は卵に対してアレルギーがあります。
    Case 2　I have metal allergy.　私は金属アレルギーがあります。

2. Have you experienced any side effects from medication?
    薬による副作用を経験したことはありますか。
    Case 1　No, I haven't.　いいえ。ありません。
    Case 2　No, I haven't.　いいえ。ありません。

3. Is there anything else that bothers you?　他に気になることはありますか。
    Case 1　My gums are swollen.　歯肉が腫れています。
    Case 2　My teeth feel loose.　歯がぐらついている感じです。

4. Do you have health insurance?　健康保険証はお持ちですか。
    Case 1　Yes, I do.　はい、持っています。
    Case 2　Yes, I do.　はい、持っています。

Lesson 6: Examination

■ 上村先生のワンポイントアドバイス ■

口腔内診察の際は何に注意するべきでしょうか。もちろん、歯科医は患者の口腔内の如何なる異常も発見しなければなりません。正常と異常を見分けるには訓練と長年の経験が必要です。

1. Core Terms

1. x-ray   2. blow   3. mirror   4. tweezers   5. appointment   6. bacteria   7. 診察   8. 歯列
9. 敏感さ   10. 歯周ポケット   11. 深さ   12. 歯垢   13. エクスプローラー   14. 歯間ブラシ

4. Core Phrases

1. 歯並びを確認します。
2. 歯に空気を吹き付けます。
3. 歯周ポケットの診査をします。
4. 歯茎の出血を確認します。
5. 虫歯のX線を撮ります。

6. Risa's Coffee Break

カルテ - patient record   →   カリエス - caries   →   アルバイト - part-time job   →   ノートパソコン - laptop computer   →   フロント - reception   →   シール - sticker   →   ペンチ - pliers   →   コンセント - outlet   →   アンケート - questionnaire   →   ギリシャ - Greece

7. Workout

1. I am going to measure the depth of the groove between your gums and teeth.
2. I will apply fluoride to your teeth.

8. Dialogs

Dialog 1

Dentist: Moshi, moshi, ...
　　　　　　　もしもし。
Bill Smith: Hello, I would like to (make) (an) (appointment).
　　　　　　　もしもし。予約を取りたいですが。
Dentist: What seems to be the problem?
　　　　　　　どうなさいましたか。
Bill Smith: My tooth hurts when I (drink) (something) (cold).
　　　　　　　冷たいものを飲むと歯が痛みます。
Dentist: OK, how about tomorrow morning?
　　　　　　　分かりました。明日の朝はいかがでしょうか。
Bill Smith: I (can't) (make) (it) in the morning. (How) (about) after 4 pm?
　　　　　　　朝は無理です。4時以降は空いていますか。
Dentist: I can fit you in at 6:30.
　　　　　　　6時半からでしたら大丈夫です。
Bill Smith: OK.
　　　　　　　それでお願いします。
Dentist: (May) (I) (have) (your) (name)?
　　　　　　　お名前は。
Bill Smith: My name is Bill Smith.
　　　　　　　ビル・スミスです。

Dentist:	All right. See you at 6:30 tomorrow evening, Mr. Smith.
	分かりました。ではスミスさん、明日の晩の6時半にお待ちしています。

Dialog 2

Dentist:	You have (plaque) (buildup) between your teeth.
	歯と歯の間に歯垢が溜まっています。
Patient:	What is plaque?
	歯垢って何ですか？
Dentist:	It is a (thin) (coating) that contains bacteria.
	細菌を含む薄い膜です。
Patient:	Is it harmful?
	それは有害ですか。
Dentist:	It may eventually lead to (cavities) and (gum) (trouble).
	やがて虫歯や歯肉のトラブルに発展するかも知れません。
Patient:	Do you think using dental floss would be effective?
	フロスを使うのは効果的でしょうか。
Dentist:	Absolutely. You may also use an (inter-dental) (brush).
	もちろん。歯間ブラシを使うのもいいですよ。

9. Listening Comprehension（巻末 Answer Sheet）

Dialog 1

Q1.　What are the symptoms?　症状は何か。
　　His tooth hurts when he drinks something cold.　冷たいものを飲んだ時に歯が痛む（しみる）。
Q2.　When is the appointment?　予約はいつなのか。
　　The appointment is at 6:30 tomorrow evening.　予約は明日の晩の6時半からである。

Dialog 2

Q1.　What is the patient's problem?　患者の状態はどうなのか。
　　He has plaque buildup between his teeth.　歯と歯の間に歯垢が溜まっている。
Q2.　What is plaque?　歯垢とは何か。
　　It is a thin coating that contains bacteria.　細菌を含む薄い膜である。
Q3.　What would be effective to remove plaque?　歯垢を取り除くのに有効なものはなにか。
　　Dental floss and inter-dental brush are effective.　フロスと歯間ブラシが有効である。

10. Test（巻末 Answer Sheet）

1. x-ray 2. appointment 3. bacteria 4. examination 5. alignment
6. sensitivity 7. periodontal pocket 8. depth 9. plaque 10. inter-dental brush

Lesson 7: Diagnosis

上村先生のワンポイントアドバイス
患者の状態を正確に診断することは良い歯科医になるための一つの条件です。口腔内の診察と同様、訓練と長年の経験で身に付きます。

1. Core Terms

1. diagnosis   2. bacterial infection   3. dry mouth   4. bad breath   5. disease   6. う蝕
7. 不適合義歯   8. 炎症   9. 脱灰   10. 歯周炎   11. 歯肉後退   12. 膿

4. Core Phrases

1. う蝕により歯に穴があいています。
2. 歯からミネラル分が失われています。
3. コーヒーとワインの飲みすぎです。
4. 長い間、歯を強く磨きすぎています。
5. 臭いの強い食べ物を食べ過ぎているのかもしれません。
6. 歯肉の病気を放置するとどうなりますか。
7. 投薬により唾液の減少が起きています。

6. Risa's Coffee Break

Question: What's this?

Answer: This is a suction. → This is a mirror. → This is an explorer. → These are tweezers. → This is an excavator.

7. Workout

1.   There is a hole in the tooth caused by decay.
     c. cavity / caries
2.   There is mineral loss from the teeth.
     e. demineralization
3.   You drink too much coffee and wine.
     a. extrinsic stains
4.   You have brushed too hard over a long period of time.
     f. receding gums
5.   You eat a lot of strong smelling food.
     d. bad breath
6.   Gum disease is left untreated.
     b. periodontitis
7.   There is a reduction of saliva due to medication.
     g. dry mouth

8. Dialogs

Dialog 1

Patient: I've been having some pain in my (upper) (right) (teeth).
          右上の歯に痛みがあります。

Dentist: Let me (blow) (some) (air) (on) them and see what is wrong.
          風を当てて確認します。

Patient: Oooh! The second one from the back is (sensitive).
          痛い。後から 2 番目の歯が敏感です。

Dentist: You either have (tooth) (decay) or some hyper-sensitivity. Open wide.
う蝕か知覚過敏ですね。大きく開けてください。

Patient: Could it be a cavity?
虫歯でしょうか。

Dentist: It sure is...and quite deep, too.
そうです。しかもかなり深いです。

Dialog 2

Patient: The area surrounding my lower back tooth (feels) (tender).
下の奥歯周辺が痛みます。

Dentist: Let's see. Open wide.
診ましょう。大きく開けてください。

Patient: So, what's wrong?
で、どうですか。

Dentist: The (gums) of your rear teeth are (swollen). Let's (take) (an) (x-ray) and check.
奥歯の周りの歯茎が腫れています。レントゲンを撮って確認しましょう。

Patient: How bad is it?
どうですか。

Dentist: As you can see here, you have pus formation and the wisdom tooth is (sideways). It is called an (impacted) (molar).
ここに見えるように、親知らずが横向きで膿が溜まっています。埋伏歯と呼びます。

[注] tender = 圧痛のある   pus formation = 化膿

9. Listening Comprehension（巻末 Answer Sheet）

Dialog 1

Q1.   What kind of symptoms does the patient have?   患者はどのような症状を訴えているか。
He has been having some pain in his upper right teeth.   右上の歯に痛みがある。

Q2.   What did the dentist do before seeing what is wrong?   歯科医は診察する前に何をしたのか。
He blew some air on the teeth.   彼は歯に空気を吹き付けた。

Q3.   What was the patient's response?   患者の反応はどうだったか。
He said it hurts.   痛みを訴えた。

Q4.   What is the diagnosis?   診断は何か。
The diagnosis is a deep cavity.   診断は深い虫歯である。

Dialog 2

Q1.   What are the patient's symptoms?   患者の症状は何か。
The area surrounding his lower back teeth feels tender.   下の奥歯の周囲が腫れています。

Q2.   What did the dentist do to check?   歯科医は確認をするために何をしたか。
He took an x-ray.   彼は X 線写真を撮った。

Q3.   What is the diagnosis?   診断の結果は。
The diagnosis is pus formation and impacted molar.   診断は智歯周囲炎です。

10. Test（巻末 Answer Sheet）

1. diagnosis 2. bacterial infection 3. dry mouth 4. bad breath 5. caries
6. inflammation 7. decalcification 8. periodontitis 9. receding gums 10. pus

Lesson 8: Treatment Procedures 2

上村先生のワンポイントアドバイス

歯の表面のわずかな凹凸や角でも不快感を引き起こします。治療そのものは歯のう蝕を取り除くことによって成功したかもしれません。しかし、研磨をきっちりしないと治療が完了したとは言えません。

1. Core Terms

1. back and forth   2. sideways   3. run   4. rough   5. うがい   6. 噛みしめる
7. ギリギリさせる   8. 凹凸や角   9. 欠ける   10. コンポジットレジン   11. 接着する   12. 磨く

4. Core Phrases

1. 歯をギリギリさせてください。   2. 少し痛みを感じるかもしれません。
3. 痛みを感じますか。   4. 舌で感触を確かめてください。
5. 凹凸や角は感じますか。

6. Risa's Coffee Break

柔らかい毛先の歯ブラシを選んでください。/ Choose a toothbrush with soft bristles.
ペンを持つように歯ブラシを持ってください。/ Hold the toothbrush with a pen grip.
歯面に対して 90 度の角度で歯ブラシを当ててください。
/ Apply the toothbrush to the surface at a 90-degree angle.
小さい動きで磨いてください。/ Brush with short strokes.
歯茎に対して 45 度の角度で歯ブラシを当ててください。
/ Apply the toothbrush to the gums at a 45-degree angle.
小さい動きで磨いてください。/ Brush with short strokes.
歯の外側、内側、そして噛む面を磨いてください。
/ Brush the outer, inner, and chewing surfaces of the teeth.
前歯の内側を磨くために歯ブラシを垂直に立ててください。
/ Tilt the brush vertically for the inside of the front teeth.

7. Workout

1. How about next Wednesday afternoon?
2. How about choosing ceramic crown? It looks natural.

8. Dialogs

Dialog 1

Dentist: What's wrong?
　　　　どうしたの。
Patient: I (tripped) and (fell) on my face.
　　　　転んで顔から落ちてしまいました。
Dentist: Oh, that's awful.
　　　　あら。それは大変だ。
Patient: I think I (broke) (my) (tooth).
　　　　歯が折れたと思います。
Dentist: Let me take a look...seems like you chipped your (upper) (incisor).
　　　　診ましょう。うーん、上顎切歯が欠けているようです。
Patient: What can be done about it?
　　　　どうすればいいでしょうか。

Dentist: Since you chipped off only a small piece, I will bond the tooth using (tooth) (colored) (composite) (resin).
少しだけ欠けていますので、歯と同じ色のレジンで埋めます。

Patient: How long will it take?
どれくらい時間がかかりますか。

Dentist: I can do it right now. It won't take long.
今すぐできます。時間はかかりません。

Dialog 2

Dentist: Try grinding your teeth (back) and (forth) and (sideways). How does it feel?
歯を前後左右にギリギリさせてください。どうですか。

Patient: It fits well.
しっくりきます。

Dentist: Could you (run) (your) (tongue) around the filling?
詰め物の周りを舌でなぞってみてください。

Patient: Yes.
はい。

Dentist: Do you feel any (bumps) or (edges)?
凹凸や角を感じますか。

Patient: The surface feels a little rough on my tongue.
表面が少しざらついているのを舌で感じます。

Dentist: O.K. I will (polish) (off) the edge. Open wide.
わかりました。角を取ります。お口を大きく開けてください。
So, how does it feel now?
どうですか。

Patient: Very smooth. Much more comfortable.
とても滑らかです。先程よりずっといいです。

Dentist: Please rinse out your mouth.
お口をすすいでください

［注］trip = つまずく

9. Listening Comprehension（巻末 Answer Sheet）

Dialog 1

Q1.   What happened to the patient?   患者に何が起きたか。
He tripped and fell on his face.   彼は転んで顔から落ちた。

Q2.   How will the dentist treat him?   歯科医はどのように治療するのか。
The dentist will bond the tooth using tooth colored composite resin.
歯と同じ色のコンポジットレジンで歯を接着する。

Dialog 2

Q1.   What did the patient feel when he ran his tongue over the filling?
患者は舌先で充填した部分を確認した時に何を感じたか。
The surface felt a little rough.   表面が少し荒いと感じた。

Q2.   What did the dentist do to solve the problem?   この問題を解決するのに歯科医は何をしたのか。
He polished off the edge.   鋭利な部分を磨いた。

Q3.   What did the patient say about the adjustment?   この調整について患者は何と言ったのか。
He said it is smooth and comfortable.   滑らかで感触がよい。

10. Test（巻末 Answer Sheet）

1. back and forth 2. sideways 3. rough 4. gargle 5. clench
6. grind 7. bumps or edges 8. composite resin 9. bond 10. polish

Lesson 9: Treating Cavities

虫歯という診断結果は患者にとってかなり衝撃的なことである。患者の気持に配慮をすることと治療を始めるよう勇気づけることが歯科医の役割です。

1. Core Terms

1. deep　　2. drill　　3. remove　　4. disinfect　　5. fill　　6. apply　　7. harden　　8. カリエス
9. 仮留め　　10. 充填　　11. 根管　　12.（削り）カス　　13. 破折　　14. 洗浄する

4. Core Phrases

1. 歯茎に局所麻酔をします。
2. 歯のう蝕に罹った部分を取り除きます。
3. 術部を消毒します。
4. 歯と同じ色の充填剤を使い光を当てます。
5. 角を削り取って磨きます。

6. Risa's Coffee Break

Question: What's this?

Answer:　This is a syringe. → This is a drill. → This is composite resin. → This is a curing light. → This is a polisher.

7. Workout

Which department should you go to?　あなたはどの教室へ行くべきか。

1. You want to know about the structure of the oral region. Which department should you go to?
   口腔領域の構造について知りたい。どこへ行くべきでしょうか。
   イ Anatomy　解剖学

2. You want to know about cell metabolism. Which department should you go to?
   細胞内代謝について知りたい。どこへ行くべきでしょか。
   エ Biochemistry　生化学

3. You want to know whether fluoride is effective or not. Which department should you go to?
   フッ化物の効果について知りたい。どこへ行くべきでしょうか。
   キ Oral Health　口腔衛生学

4. You want to know how saliva is secreted. Which department should you go to?
   唾液の分泌について知りたい。どこへ行くべきでしょうか。
   カ Physiology　生理学

5. You want to know the different properties of metals. Which department should you go to?
   金属の色んな特性について知りたい。どこへ行くべきでしょうか。
   ク Dental Materials　歯科理工学

6. You want to know about Streptococcus mutans. Which department should you go to?
   ミュタンス連鎖菌について知りたい。どこへ行くべきでしょうか。
   ウ Bacteriology　細菌学

7. You want to know how drugs are effective. Which department should you go to?
   薬の効果について知りたい。どこへ行くべきでしょうか。
   ア Pharmacology　薬理学

8. You want to know the mechanism of oral diseases. Which department should you go to?
   口腔内の病気のメカニズムについて知りたい。どこへ行くべきでしょうか。
   オ Pathology　病理学

8. Dialogs

Dialog 1

Dentist: What's wrong?
どうされましたか。

Patient: My (lower) (back) (tooth) hurts...on the right side.
下の奥歯が痛いです。右側です。

Dentist: Since when?
いつからですか。

Patient: It started a few days ago. But now I (can't) (stand) (it).
数日前からです。しかし今は我慢できません。

Dentist: Let's see. Open wide. You have a big cavity in your (lower) (first) (molar). Let's take an x-ray for more detail.
診ましょう。大きく開けてください。下の第一大臼歯に大きなう蝕があります。レントゲンを撮って詳しく見ましょう。

Dentist: As this image on the monitor shows, the cavity is quite deep and the (dental) (pulp) (is) (affected).
モニターの画像が示しているように、う蝕はかなり深く、歯髄に達しています。

Patient: Oh no. What needs to be done?
参ったな。どうすればいいですか。

Dentist: I suggest we do (root) (canal) (treatment).
根管治療をお勧めします。

Patient: Starting now?
今からですか。

Dentist: Today, I will put a (temporary) (filling) in to stop the pain. We will start the treatment in a couple of days.
今日は仮封をして痛みを止めます。数日後に治療を始めます。

Dialog 2

Dentist: Look at the x-ray. The discolored area shows (the) (extent) (of) (decay).
レントゲン画像を見てください。変色した部分がう蝕の範囲を示しています。

Patient: Is it serious?
深刻ですか。

Dentist: I'm afraid so. It has (infected) (the) (nerve). You will need root canal treatment.
残念ながらそうです。歯髄が感染しています。根管治療が必要です。

Patient: What are you going to do?
どのようなことをするのですか。

Dentist: I will (drill) (out) the decayed area. Then I will disinfect the root canal. Finally, I will fill the tooth and (cover) it with a metal crown.
う蝕の部分を削り取ります。次に根管を消毒します。最後に詰めてメタルクラウンを被せます。

Patient: Will it be painful?
痛みますか。

Dentist: Don't worry. There will be (less) (pain) than now.
心配しないでください。今よりは痛みが減ります。

Patient: How many visits will it take?
何回来ないといけませんか。

Dentist: I would say about 5 or 6 visits.
5、6回ですかね。

9. Listening Comprehension （巻末 Answer Sheet）

Dialog 1

Q1.   What symptoms is the patient complaining about?   患者はどのような症状を訴えているのか。
　　　His lower back tooth on the right hurts.   右下の奥歯が痛む。

Q2.   What is the result of the x-ray?   X 線撮影の結果わかったことは何か。
　　　The cavity is deep and the pulp is affected.   虫歯が深く、歯髄が侵されている。

Q3.   What kind of treatment did the dentist suggest?   歯科医はどのような治療を提案したか。
　　　The dentist suggests root canal treatment.   歯科医は根管治療を提案した。

Dialog 2

Q1.   Why does the patient need root canal treatment?   患者はなぜ根管治療が必要なのか。
　　　The decay has infected the nerve.   う蝕が歯髄に達している。

Q2.   What is the procedure of the treatment?   治療の手順は何か。
　　　He will drill out the decayed area. Then he will disinfect the root canal. Finally, he will fill the tooth and cover it with a metal crown.
　　　う蝕の部分を削り取る。次に根管を消毒する。最後に充填をしてメタルクラウンを被せる。

Q3.   How does the dentist explain about the pain of the treatment?
　　　歯科医は治療中の痛みについてどのように説明しているのか。
　　　There will be less pain than now.   今よりは痛みは少ない。

10. Test （巻末 Answer Sheet）

1. deep 2. drill 3. disinfect 4. fill 5. caries   6. temporary filling 7. permanent filling 8. root canal
9. fracture 10. cleanse

Lesson 10: Prosthetics

上村先生のワンポイントアドバイス

我々の社会はますますデジタル化されています。近い将来、手で印象材を混ぜて素早くトレーに盛り付けるのは時代遅れになるかもしれません。しかし、いくら技術が進歩してもこのような基本的な作業は重要であり、我々の教育として残すべきです。

1. Core Terms

1. adjust 2. metal 3. ceramic 4. fit 5. natural 6. match 7. place 8. 接着剤 9. 審美的な
10. 陶材 11. 色調 12. 咬合 13. 印象 14. 粘状のもの

4. Core Phrases

1. どの種類のクラウンになさいますか。
2. 周囲の歯と合う色を選んでください。
3. このシェイドガイドを見てください。
4. まず装着の具合を確認します。
5. 次に噛み合わせを確認します。
6. 最後に接着剤でクラウンをつけます。
7. 入れ歯用ブラシを使って食べかすを取り除いてください。
8. 入れ歯をぬるま湯ですすいでください。

6. Risa's Coffee Break

適量のアルジネート印象材と水を使う。水を入れてヘラで混ぜ始める。ボウルの側面を使い、ダマや気泡を取り除く。滑らかになるまで混ぜる。トレーに盛り付ける。
1. alginate 2. bowl 3. measuring cup 4. tray 5. spatula

7. Workout

1. My back tooth is growing sideways and needs to be extracted.
   奥歯が横向きで抜歯の必要があります。 Oral Surgery　口腔外科
2. My cavity seems very deep. It is causing severe pain.
   虫歯が深いようです。激しい痛みを引き起こしています。 Endodontics　歯内治療科
3. My teeth alignment is crowded.
   歯並びが悪いです。 Orthodontics　歯科矯正科
4. My gums are swollen and bleeding.
   歯肉が腫れて出血しています。 Periodontics　歯周病科
5. I want artificial teeth that feel like my own.
   自分の歯のような差し歯が欲しいです。 Implantology　インプラント科
6. Recently, my bridge doesn't seem to fit right.
   最近ブリッジがしっくりしません。 Prosthodontics　補綴科
7. I need to have my cavity treated.
   虫歯の治療をする必要があります。 Operative Dentistry　保存科
8. My child has tooth trouble.
   子供の歯に問題があります。 Pediatric Dentistry　小児歯科
9. My grandma's dentures are missing.
   おばあちゃんの入れ歯が見当たらない。 Geriatric Dentistry　高齢者歯科

8. Dialogs

Dialog 1

Dentist: I will (take) (an) (impression) with this tray filled with rubbery substance.
この印象材の入っているトレーで型取りをします。

Patient: Oh, I hate this. It makes me gag.
これは嫌だな。おえっとなるよ。

Dentist: Just try and hold on (for) (about) (a) (minute).
1分間ほど頑張ってください。

Patient: O.K. I'll try my best.
わかった。頑張ります。

Dentist: We are finished. You may (rinse) (out) your mouth now.
お疲れ様でした。お口をすすいでください。

Patient: So, what's next?
次は何ですか。

Dentist: I am going to put in a (temporary) (crown). We'll be ready to (place) and (adjust) the permanent crown a week from now.
仮歯を入れます。被せものは1週間後にできてきます。

Patient: In the (meantime), can I eat as usual?
その間は、普通に食事をしてもいいでしょうか。

Dentist: Be careful with (hard) or (sticky) food. Also, try to chew (on) (the) (other) (side).
固いものや引っ付きやすいものには注意してください。また、反対側で噛むようにしてください。

Dialog 2

Patient: I'm not sure. Which should I choose? (Porcelain) or (metal)?
どちらを選んだらいいのかな。陶材それとも金属。

Dentist: I think metal will do. It is stronger and I won't have to (drill) (away) too much of the (remaining) (tooth). On top of that, your (insurance) will only cover a metal one.
金属がよいと思います。強い上に、もとの歯をそれほど削らなくてもいいのです。さらに、金属の場合は、保険が利きます。

Patient: Wouldn't it look bad (esthetically)?
見た目は悪くありませんか。

Dentist: Since the cavity is in the rear, it won't be (visible) ... unless you open your mouth very wide.
後ろにあるため見えませんよ。お口を大きく開けない限りは。

Patient: Like when I yawn?
あくびをする時ですか。

Dentist: But people cover their mouths, don't they?
でも普通は、手で口を隠しますよね。

［注］gag＝えづく　yawn＝あくび

9. Listening Comprehension （巻末 Answer Sheet）

Dialog 1

Q1. Why is the patient reluctant to take an impression?　患者はなぜ印象材を嫌がっているのか。
It makes him gag.　えづくから。

Q2. What kind of treatment will the dentist do for that day?
歯科医師はその日、どのような治療をするのか。
The dentist will put in a temporary crown.　歯科医は仮歯を入れる。

Q3. What should the patient be careful of?　患者は何に注意をするべきか。
He should be careful with hard or sticky food.　硬い食べ物や歯に引っ付く食べ物に注意するべき。

Dialog 2

Q1.　What are the three reasons why the dentist recommends a metal crown?

歯科医がメタルクラウンを勧める 3 つの理由は何か。

Metal crowns are stronger. Also, there is no need to drill away too much of the remaining tooth. And, they are covered by insurance.

メタルクラウンの方が強い。また、元の歯をそれほど削る必要がないから。そして、保険適用であるから。

Q2.　What is the patient worried about concerning metal crowns?

患者はメタルクラウンについて何が心配なのか。

They look bad esthetically.　　見た目が悪い。

Q3.　Why does the dentist think the patient's worry is not a problem?

なぜ歯科医は患者の心配していることは問題ではないと考えているのか。

People cover their mouths when they yawn.　人々はあくびの際に手で口を隠す。

10. Test（巻末 Answer Sheet）

1. adjust 2. metal 3. ceramic 4. natural 5. place 6. esthetic 7. porcelain 8. shade 9. occlusion
10. impression

Lesson 11: Gum Trouble / Gum Disease

虫歯同様、歯周病は日々のセルフケアで予防することができる。市場には多くのセルフ
ケア商品があります。しかし、最も重要なのは、正しくセルフケアを行うための歯科医
による指導である。

1. Core Terms

1. infection   2. suffer from   3. tendency   4. improper   5. reaction   6. 歯肉
7. スケーリング   8. 痛い   9. 歯石   10. 歯周病   11. 後退する

4. Core Phrases

1. 糖尿病患者は歯周病を患う傾向がある。
2. 歯肉の後退は不適切な歯磨きにより引き起こされる。
3. 上の前歯がぐらつく感じである。
4. 歯茎の赤味は炎症の症状の一つである。
5. 膿は細菌感染に対するあなたの歯肉の反応である。

6. Risa's Coffee Break

Question: What's this?

Answer: This is a <u>toothbrush</u>. / This is an <u>inter-dental brush</u>. / This is <u>toothpaste</u>. / This is <u>dental floss</u>.
/ This is a <u>scaler</u>.

8. Dialogs

Dialog 1

A: What did you (have) (for) (lunch) today?
今日の昼ごはん、何食べた。

B: A bowl of clam chowder and some rolls, why?
クラムチャウダーとロールパンだが、どうしたの。

A: Your breath (smells) (strongly) (of) onions.
息が玉ねぎの臭いのようだ。

B: Strange. I didn't have any.
変だな、食べていないが。

A: Maybe (something) is (wrong) (with) your gums.
もしかしたら歯茎に何かが起きているかも。

B: Really?
本当か？

A: Yes, I noticed they look swollen and a bit discolored.
そう。腫れている上に少し色も悪いよ。

Dialog 2

Patient: My gums have been feeling (a) (bit) (sore) lately.
最近、歯茎が少し痛いです。

Dentist: Let's see what is going on. Open wide.... There is (some) (bleeding) from your gums.
どうなっているか診ましょう。お口を大きく開けてください。歯茎から少し出血しています。

Patient: Why is that happening?
原因は何ですか。

Dentist: (It) (is) (caused) (by) infection. I will do some cleaning and disinfect it.
感染が原因です。きれいにして消毒しておきます。

Dialog 3

Dentist: You seem to have (tartar) (buildup).
        歯石が付いています。

Patient: Is it bad?
        状態は悪いですか。

Dentist: Yes, especially (behind) your lower front teeth. It is causing the (swelling) (of) your gums.
        そうですね。特に下の前歯の裏側にたまっています。それが歯茎の腫れを引き起こしています。

Patient: How will you treat it?
        どのように治療しますか。

Dentist: My (hygienist) will remove the tartar with an (ultrasonic) (scaler).
        衛生士さんが超音波スケーラーで歯石を取り除きます。

Patient: Will it hurt?
        痛みますか。

Dentist: Just in case, I will spread some anesthetic around the (sensitive) parts.
        痛みに備えて感じやすいところには表面麻酔を行います。

［注］buildup = 堆積

9. Listening Comprehension（巻末 Answer Sheet）

Dialog 1

Q1.　What is wrong with the man's breath?　　男性の息にどのような問題があるのか。
　　His breath smells strongly of onions.　　彼の息は玉ねぎのような匂いが強くする。

Q2.　How do his gums appear?　　彼の歯茎はどのように見えるのか。
　　They look swollen and a bit discolored.　　腫れて少し色が悪いように見える。

Dialog 2

Q1.　What is the patient's complaint?　　患者は何を訴えているのか。
　　His gums have been feeling a bit sore lately.　　最近歯茎が少し痛む。

Q2.　What did the dentist see inside the patient's mouth?　　歯科医は患者の口の中に何を確認したか。
　　There is some bleeding from the gums.　　歯茎から少し出血がある。

Q3.　How will the condition be treated?　　どのような処置を行うのか。
　　The dentist will clean and disinfect the site.　　歯科医は患部の洗浄と消毒を行う。

Dialog 3

Q1.　What is the patient's problem?　　患者は何で困っているのか。
　　He has tartar buildup behind the lower front teeth. It is causing the swelling of his gums.
　　下の前歯の裏に歯石が蓄積している。これが歯茎の腫れを引き起こしている。

Q2.　What kind of treatment will be conducted?　　どのような治療が行われるのか。
　　The tartar will be removed with an ultrasonic scaler.　　超音波スケーラーで歯石を取り除く。

Q3.　What precaution will be taken?　　どのような予防策が取られるのか。
　　Some anesthetic will be spread around the sensitive parts.　　敏感な部分に麻酔薬を塗る。

10. Test（巻末 Answer Sheet）

1. infection 2. suffer from 3. tendency 4. improper 5. reaction 6. gingiva 7. scaling 8. sore
9. calculus 10. periodontal disease

Lesson 12: Oral Care Habits

上村先生のワンポイントアドバイス
患者がお口の手入れをどのようにしているか正しく理解することは治療の結果にも影響を与える。たとえ間違ったことをしていても決して批判をしてはいけません。むしろ患者を動機づけて一緒に「よりよい」手入の方法を考えるようにしましょう。

1. Core Terms
1. brush　　2. brushing　　3. meal　　4. supplement　　5. floss　　6. warn　　7. お口のお手入れ
8. 洗口液　　9. 投薬　　10. ウオーターピック

4. Core Phrases
1. いつ歯を磨きますか。
2. 1回あたりの歯磨きにかける時間はどれくらいですか。
3. 歯磨き以外にお口のお手入れはされていますか。
4. タバコは吸いますか。
5. 平均の睡眠時間はどれくらいですか。
6. 間食はしますか。
7. 現在何かの治療を受けていますか。
8. お薬を服用していますか。

6. Risa's Coffee Break
ダンボール - cardboard　→ フライドポテト – French fries　→ ワクチン - vaccine　→
カンニング - cheating　→ ウィルス - virus　→ シャーペン – mechanical pencil　→
デッドボール – hit by pitch　→ ジェットコースター – roller coaster　→
スイス - Switzerland　→ ペットボトル – plastic bottle

7. Workout
1. An appointment is available from 5 pm.
2. A hygienist is available tomorrow afternoon.

8. Dialogs
Case 1
Q1: When do you brush your teeth?
いつ歯を磨きますか。
A:　(After) (each) (meal).
毎食後。
Q2: How much time do you spend on each brushing?
毎回どれくらい時間をかけますか。
A:　(About) (three) (minutes).
約3分。
Q3: Do you have any other oral care habits besides brushing?
歯磨き以外にお手入れはしていますか。
A:　I (rinse) (with) mouthwash.
洗口液で口をすすぎます。
Q4: Do you smoke?
タバコは吸いますか。
A:　No, (not) (any) (more).
いいえ。もう吸っていません。

Q5: How many hours of sleep do you get on average?
平均の睡眠時間はどれくらいですか。

A: About (six) (or) (seven) hours.
約6, 7時間。

Q6: What do you usually drink?
普段は何をよく飲みますか。

A: I constantly drink coffee (throughout) (the) (day). I also have some wine at dinner time.
1日中コーヒーを飲んでいます。夕食時にワインも少し飲みます。

Q7: Do you eat between meals?
間食はしますか。

A: Sometimes I munch on a bag of potato chips.
時々ポテトチップスを食べています。

Q8: Are you receiving any medical treatment now?
治療中のご病気はありますか。

A: No, I'm not.
いいえ。

Q9: Are you taking any medication?
薬は服用していますか。

A: (Besides) various supplements, no.
幾つかのサプリ以外は服用していません。

Case 2

Q1: When do you brush your teeth?
いつ歯を磨きますか。

A: In the (morning) and (before) (bedtime).
朝と就寝前です。

Q2: How much time do you spend on each brushing?
毎回どれくらい時間をかけますか。

A: (A) (couple) (of) (minutes) for brushing and then I floss.
歯磨きに数分。その後フロスをします。

Q3: Do you do anything else besides brushing?
歯磨き以外にお手入れはしていますか。

A: I use (dental) (floss) and sometimes a (water) (pick).
フロスと時々ウォーターピックを使います。

Q4: Do you smoke?
タバコは吸いますか。

A: Yes, about (a) (pack) (a) (day).
はい。1日1箱くらいです。

Q5: How many hours of sleep do you get on average?
平均の睡眠時間はどれくらいですか。

A: I've been losing sleep because of my busy schedule. I guess about 5 hours (at) (the) (most).
忙しくて寝不足です。多くて5時間くらいです。

Q6: What do you usually drink?
普段は何をよく飲みますか。

A: I drink (a) (lot) (of) mineral water. I also like to drink coke.
ミネラルウォーターをよく飲みます。またコーラも好きです。

Q7: Do you eat between meals?
間食はしますか。

A: No, I don't.
いいえ。

Q8: Are you receiving any medical treatment now?
　　治療中のご病気はありますか。
A:　No, but my doctor (warned) (me) (about) my high blood pressure.
　　医者から高血圧に注意するように言われています。
Q9: Are you taking any medication?
　　薬は服用していますか。
A:　I am (taking) (medication) (for) my blood pressure.
　　血圧の薬を服用しています。

9. Practice（巻末 Answer Sheet）

Case 1

Q1: When do you brush your teeth?
　　I brush my teeth after each meal.　　毎食後に歯を磨いています。
Q2: How much time do you spend on each brushing?
　　I spend about 5 minutes on each brushing.　　それぞれの歯磨きに5分ほどかけます。
Q3: Do you have any other oral care habits besides brushing?
　　I use mouthwash.　　洗口液を使います。
Q4: Do you smoke?
　　No, I don't.　　いいえ。
Q5: How many hours of sleep do you get on average?
　　I would say about 6 hours.　　6時間ほどですかね。
Q6: What do you usually drink?
　　I am a serious coffee drinker!　　私はコーヒー愛好家です。
Q7: Do you eat between meals?
　　I love jellybeans.　　ジェリービーンズが大好きです。
Q8: Are you receiving any medical treatment now?
　　I am seeing my doctor for diabetes.　　糖尿病で医者へ通っています。
Q9: Are you taking any medication?
　　Yes, what my doctor prescribes.　　医者が処方する薬を。

10. Role Playing（巻末 Answer Sheet）

Case 2

Q1: When do you brush your teeth?
　　解答例 :I brush my teeth in the morning and evening.　　朝と晩に歯を磨いています。
Q2: How much time do you spend on each brushing?
　　解答例 :Three to four minutes.　　3〜4分。
Q3: Do you have any other oral care habits besides brushing?
　　解答例 :I sometimes use mouthwash.　　時々洗口液を使います。
Q4: Do you smoke?
　　解答例 :Yes, I do. I smoke 2 or 3 cigarettes a day.　　はい。1日2〜3本を吸います。
Q5: How many hours of sleep do you get on average?
　　解答例 :I get about 7 hours of sleep.　　7時間ほどです。
Q6: What do you usually drink?
　　解答例 :I love orange juice.　　オレンジジュースが大好きです。
Q7: Do you eat between meals?
　　解答例 :Yes, I do. I eat cookies.　　はい。クッキーを食べます。
Q8: Are you receiving any medical treatment now?
　　解答例 :No, I am not.　　いいえ、受けていません。
Q9: Are you taking any medication?
　　解答例 :No, I am not.　　いいえ、服用していません。

Lesson 13: Giving Advice

上村先生のワンポイントアドバイス　治療が終わると患者は帰宅後の指示を待っています。いつから食事をしていいか、いつ頃痛みが引くかなど十分な情報を与える必要があります。気になることは何でも質問するように伝えます。また問題がある時はいつでも電話をするようにとも伝えます。これは、大切なことです。

1. Core Terms

1. toothpaste　2. avoid　3. pill　4. surface　5. follow　6. regular　7. フッ化物
8. 柔らかい毛先　9. 歯間ブラシ　10. 痛み止め　11. 抗生剤　12. 軟膏　13. 処方する
14. 処方箋　15. 念のため

4. Core Phrases

1. 固い食べ物は避けてください。
2. 左側では噛まないでください。
3. 治療した歯で噛まないでください。
4. 何かありましたらお電話してください。
5. 必ず処方箋に従ってください。
6. 1回1錠を1日3回毎食後に服用してください。

6. Risa's Coffee Break

う蝕になりかけている。The decay is about to start.
エナメル質がう蝕にかかっている。The enamel is decayed.
う蝕が象牙質にすすんでいる。The decay has advanced to the dentin.
歯髄が侵されている。The pulp has been affected.
歯根のみが残っている。Only the roots of the tooth remain.

7. Workout

1. You may not eat or drink for one hour.
2. To prevent stains, please refrain from smoking.

8. Dialogs

Dialog 1
Patient: How should I brush my teeth correctly?
どのようにすれば正しく歯を磨けますか。
Dentist: Since your gums are (sensitive), be sure to use a toothbrush with (soft) (bristles).
歯茎が敏感になっているため毛先の柔らかい歯ブラシを使ってください。
Patient: (What) (about) toothpaste?
歯磨き粉は。
Dentist: Don't use too much. Regular toothpaste (should) (be) (fine).
あまり使いすぎないでください。普通のもので大丈夫です。
Patient: Am I brushing too hard?
強く磨きすぎですか。
Dentist: (I) (am) (afraid) (so). Brush softly as if you are raking leaves off the surface of a rock garden.
残念ながらそうです。石庭の落ち葉をそっと集めるように磨いてください。
Patient: Wow! That sounds poetic.
すごい！まるで詩のようだ。

Dialog 2

Dentist: I have (placed) a temporary filling in the cavity.
治療したところに仮留めを入れました。

Patient: When can I start eating?
いつから食事ができますか。

Dentist: Be sure to wait (at) (least) 30 minutes.
少なくとも 30 分は待ってください。

Patient: Would it (be) (alright) (to) eat hard food such as almonds?
アーモンドのような固い食べものは食べてもいいですか。

Dentist: Sure, as long as you (don't) (chew) (on) the right side.
いいですよ。右側で噛まないかぎりは。

Patient: Will it start hurting again?
また痛み出しますか。

Dentist: I don't think so, but I have prescribed some (pain) (killers), (antibiotics), and (mouthwash) just in case.
大丈夫だと思いますが、念のために、痛み止めと抗生剤と洗口液を処方しておきました。

［注］rake ＝ 熊手でかく

9. Listening Comprehension （巻末 Answer Sheet）

Dialog 1

Q1. What kind of toothbrush is recommended?   どのような歯ブラシがお勧めか。
A toothbrush with soft bristles is recommended.   柔らかい毛先の歯ブラシがお勧めである。

Q2. What about toothpaste?   どのような歯磨き粉がお勧めか。
Regular toothpaste is recommended.   普通の歯磨き粉がお勧めである。

Q3. How should the patient brush?   患者はどのように歯を磨くべきか。
The patient should brush softly (as if raking leaves off the surface of a rock garden).
患者はそっと磨くべきである（石庭の表面から落ち葉をかき取るように）。

Dialog 2

Q1. What precautions should the patient take?   患者は何に注意するべきか。
The patient should not chew on the right side.   患者は右側で噛まないようにするべきである。

Q2. What did the dentist prescribe, just in case?   念のために歯科医は何を処方したか。
He prescribed some pain killers, antibiotics, and mouthwash.
彼は痛み止めと抗生剤と洗口液を処方した。

10. Test （巻末 Answer Sheet）

1. toothpaste 2. avoid 3. surface 4. fluoride 5. soft bristles 6. pain killer 7. antibiotics
8. ointment 9. prescribe 10. prescription

Lesson 14: Payment and Appointment

歯科治療において時間の管理は特に重要です。例えば次回の予約を決める時に補綴物を準備するのに必要な時間を考慮しなければなりません。一方で時間が空きすぎると補綴物が入らなくなることもあります。

1. Core Terms

1. cash only   2. accept   3. credit card   4. cancel   5. convenient   6. later
7. 支払い   8. 請求書   9. 延期   10. 受付   11. 合計金額   12. 利用可能   13. 道順

4. Core Phrases

1. 道順を教えてください。
2. まっすぐ進んで中華料理屋のところで左に曲がってください。
3. 次の予約はいつにされますか。
4. ご都合のよい時間は。
5. 来週の土曜日の 5 時はいかがでしょうか。
6. 5:30 も空いています。

6. Risa's Coffee Break

始めましょうか。Shall we start? お待たせしてすみません。Sorry to keep you waiting.
お大事に。Take care. ではまた次回に。See you next time.
1 分間じっとしてください。Hold still for a minute.

7. Workout

抗菌薬 antimicrobial drug
1 回 1 錠を毎食後に 3 日間飲んでください。
Take (one) tablet (three) (times) (a) (day) after each meal.
必ず飲み切ってください。
Be (sure) (to) (finish) all the medicine.

鎮痛剤 pain killer
痛みが出た場合はその都度 1 錠ずつ飲んでください。
Take (one) tablet (when) you have pain.

含嗽薬（がんそうやく）mouthwash
抜歯したあとの傷口が治るまでの間、1 日数回口の中を消毒してください。
(Rinse) (with) mouthwash (several) (times) (a) (day) until the extraction site heals.

ステロイド steroids
口内炎の患部に 1 日数回塗布してください。
(Apply) (to) the canker sore several times a day.

抗ヘルペスウイルス薬 anti-herpesvirus drug
5 日間、1 日 1 回食後に服用してください。
Take one tablet a day for five days (after) (meals).

8. Dialogs

Dialog 1
Receptionist: Mr. Parker?
　　　　　　　パーカーさん。
Patient:　　　Yes.
　　　　　　　はい。

Receptionist: (Here) (is) (your) bill.
こちらが請求書になります。

Patient: Is this covered by my Kokuminhoken, my (National) (Health) (Insurance)?
これは国民保険の範囲ですよね。

Receptionist: Yes, it is. You pay (thirty) (percent) of the total cost.
そうです。総額の 30% をお支払いいただきます。

Patient: So, how much is it?
いくらになりますか。

Receptionist: It all comes to (2200) (yen).
合計 2200 円になります。

Patient: Do you accept credit card?
クレジットカードは使えますか。

Receptionist: Yes, we do.
はい。

Dialog 2

Receptionist: When can you come for the next treatment?
次回はいつ来れますか。

Patient: I can come (on) (Wednesday) and (Friday) (evenings).
水曜日と金曜日の晩に来られます。

Receptionist: What time would be convenient?
何時頃がよろしいですか。

Patient: (The) (later) (the) (better).
遅ければ遅いほどいいです。

Receptionist: How about Friday next week at 7 pm?
来週の金曜日、7 時からはいかがですか。

Patient: Do you have anything later than that?
それよりも遅い時間はありますか。

Receptionist: Well, 7:30 (is) also (available).
7:30 でしたら空いています。

Patient: O.K. I would like to (make) (an) (appointment) at that time.
ではその時間に予約します。

9. Listening Comprehension（巻末 Answer Sheet）

Dialog 1

Q1. What kind of insurance does the patient have?   患者はどのような保険に加入しているのか。
He has National Health Insurance.   彼は国民保険に加入している。

Q2. What percentage must he pay?   彼は何割を負担するのか。
He must pay 30%.   彼は 3 割を負担しなければならない。

Q3. How will he pay?   彼はどのように払うのか。
He will pay by credit card.   彼はクレジットカードで支払う。

Dialog 2

Q1. When will the next appointment be?   次の予約はいつなのか。
The next appointment will be Friday next week at 7:30.
次の予約は次週の金曜日 7 時半からである。

10. Test（巻末 Answer Sheet）

1. cash only 2. accept 3. convenient 4. payment 5. bill 6. postpone 7. reception 8. total cost
9. available 10. directions

QRコードで動画が見られる!

歯科医学英語ワークブック

第2版

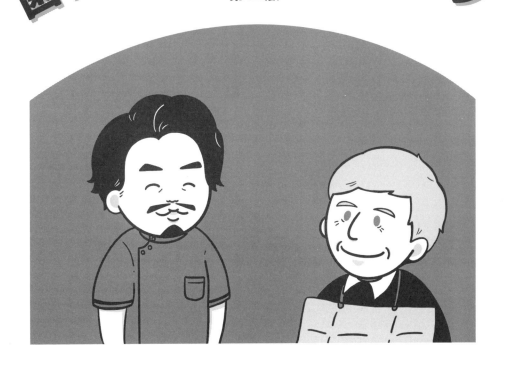

[著者]　藤田 淳一　　Brian Bachman

　　　　岡　隼人　　　Bernard MacMugen

　　　　上村 直也　　穴田 理嵯

　　　　岡村 友玄　　石原 里紗

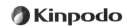

はじめに

　ある日のこと、突然歯科医の友人から電話がかかってきました。急患の外国人が来院したため通訳をしてくれないかという内容でした。お子様が転倒して歯（永久歯）が欠けたらしく、大変心配な様子でした。親子とも日本語が話せない上に、友人は英語が苦手なため、患者さんの不安がさらに大きくなっていたようです。その時に行ったスカイプによる通訳は、処置の説明、今後のケアの仕方、薬の飲み方など内容が多岐にわたりました。言葉が通じたため、親子はそれまでとは一変して非常に安心したようです。来日して一番満足のいく治療だったという嬉しいメッセージが後日届きました。

　日本に在住する外国人は年々増加しています。これに合わせて歯科医院を訪れる外国人患者も増えることが想像できます。上記のようなスカイプ通訳は、患者及び歯科医師双方にとって大変心強い味方となるでしょう。しかし、理想を言えば、歯科医師や歯科衛生士自身が直接英語で外国人患者とコミュニケーションをとることです。

　そこで我々は、歯科医及びスタッフが通訳を介さずに直接英語で対応できることを目指して本テキストを作成しました。歯学部や衛生士学校等の授業で学ぶ様々な専門用語（technical terms）はもちろん重要です。しかし歯科に関して素人である外国人患者が理解するためには一般的な用語（lay terms）も重要です。本テキストは一般用語と専門用語を織り交ぜながら初学者が無理なく単語やフレーズを覚えられるようにワークブック形式になっています。歯科医、歯科衛生士、歯科技工を目指す学生さんから歯科医院のスタッフの方々まで広く活用していただけるテキストです。

【改訂版の出版に際して】

　大学用に出版されている英語教材の音声や映像は、付録のCDやDVDで提供されているケースがほとんどです。しかし、ラジカセやプレーヤーを所有している学生は少なく、せっかくの音声教材が無駄になっています。本書では、スマートフォンでQRコードを読み取って動画を視聴します。それにより、Wi-Fi環境さえあれば、いつ、どこでも歯科医学英語の勉強をすることができます。また、すべての動画にPCからアクセスできるようURLも用意しています。LL教室やPC教室などでの授業、またより大きい画面で視聴したい方に使っていただければと思います。

2020年4月

著者代表　藤田　淳一

i

【著者紹介】

- 藤田淳一（ふじた　じゅんいち）大阪歯科大学英語教室
- 岡隼人（おか　はやと）大阪歯科大学英語教室
- 上村直也（うえむら　なおや）大阪歯科大学口腔インプラント学講座（非常勤講師）歯科医師
- 岡村友玄（おかむら　ともはる）大阪歯科大学口腔病理学講座　歯科医師
- 穴田理嵯（あなだ　りさ）大阪歯科大学OB　歯科医師
- 石原里紗（いしはら　りさ）大阪歯科大学OB　歯科医師
- Brian Bachman（ブライアン　バックマン）大阪歯科大学英語教室（非常勤講師）
- Bernard MacMugen（バーナード　マックムーゲン）大阪歯科大学英語教室（非常勤講師）

Illustrations by noriko
Special thanks to DjD (The Disc Jockey of Dentistry) and Dr. Yu Mikami
撮影協力：医療法人 上村歯科

Contents

Lesson 1   Treatment Procedures　診療にともなう動作 ································ 1

Lesson 2   General Terms　一般的な用語 ······························· 5

Lesson 3   Parts of the Mouth　各部の名称 ·························· 9

　　　　　　DJD interview program Dr. Naoya Uemura ············ 13

Lesson 4   Interview　問診に必要な用語 ····························· 15

Lesson 5   Interview 2　問診に必要な用語 ·························· 19

Lesson 6   Examination　診察 ···································· 23

　　　　　　DJD interview program Dr. Yu Mikami ·············· 27

Lesson 7   Diagnosis　診断 ······································ 29

Lesson 8   Treatment Procedures 2　診療にともなう動作 ········· 33

Lesson 9   Treating Cavities　虫歯 ······························· 37

　　　　　　DJD interview program Mr. Brian Bachman ·········· 41

Lesson 10   Prosthetics　補綴物 ··································· 43

Lesson 11   Gum Trouble / Gum Disease　歯肉炎 ················ 47

Lesson 12   Oral Care Habits　オーラルケア習慣 ················· 51

Lesson 13   Giving Advice　患者への指導 ························· 59

　　　　　　DJD interview program Dr. Naoya Uemura again ······ 57

Lesson 14   Payment and Appointment　支払いと次回の予約 ······ 63

Answer Sheet（Lesson 1〜14）

別冊：回答集

本書の使い方

動画へのアクセス
スマートフォンにQRコードリーダーなどのアプリが事前にインストールされているか確認してください。スマートフォンでテキスト内に印刷されているQRコードを読み取ります。パスワード（2020）を入力していただきますと、そのレッスンの動画がまとめて表示されます。必要な動画を選んで再生してください。以下のURLにテキスト内のすべての動画があります。▶ https://vimeo.com/showcase/lesson1-14

上村先生のワンポイントアドバイス
上村先生が歯科医として日頃心掛けていること、歯学部生時代のこと、英語の勉強で気付いたことなどを英語でアドバイスしています。レッスン前に軽く読んで頭を「英語モード」に切り替えましょう。

1　Core Terms
各レッスンのテーマに関連する用語です。これらの用語を英語及び日本語に訳して空所に書き込みます。授業では、学生同士でペアを組みます。片方の学生は、テキストを見ながら各用語を読み上げます。もう一方の学生は、それに対して（テキストを見ず）素早く英語又は日本語に訳します。この練習方法をQuick Responseと呼び、英単語を目ではなく、耳で覚える練習です。

2　Brian's Pronunciation Practice （動画付き）
Core Termsで取り上げられた単語をブライアン先生が発音します。動画を見ながら彼に続いて発音の練習をしましょう。

3　Bernie's Pronunciation Tips （動画付き）
日本人が特に苦手としている発音に焦点を当て、バーニー先生がゆっくりと発話しています。動画を見て、下線部の発音に注意しながら、彼に続いてリピートしましょう。

4　Core Phrases
各レッスンのテーマに関連するフレーズです。Core Termsを含んでいます。ここではきっちりと日本語に訳す練習をします。

5　Quick Response （動画付き）
Core PhrasesのフレーズでQuick Responseの練習をします。動画を見ながらリサ先生の日本語に対する英訳を瞬時に言います。今までの英語の勉強は文字を見て覚えてきました。しかし、実

際に外国人患者の対応をするときは、文字を当てにすることはできません。相手が発した英語を聞いて即座に反応しなければなりません。そこで通訳者の養成教育によく用いられるクィックレスポンスの練習をします。動画で読み上げられた日本語を聞いて即座に英語に訳す練習です。ポイントは動画の音声に対して即座に反応することです。Lesson 2のみフレーズではなく単語の Quick Response になっています。

6　Risa's Coffee Break（動画付き）
歯科医院で使われる器具を英語でどういうか、リサ先生の問いかけに対してバーニー先生とブライアン先生が教えてくれます。他にカタカナ英語の正しい言い方や歯科医院内の各部屋の呼び方などの問いかけがあります。動画に合わせて発音してください。

7　Workout（一部動画付き）
歯科英語についての知識をさらに深めるコーナーです。

8　Dialogs（動画付き）
歯科医院での外国人患者の対応で起こりそうな場面を対話形式の動画にしています。まず動画を見て概要を理解してください。その後、再び動画を見ながらテキスト内の空欄を埋めます。

9　Listening Comprehension
Dialogs の対話文の理解を深めるための練習です。8の動画をもう一度見て、巻末の内容に関する質問に答えます。その際、テキスト中の対話文は見ずに動画の視聴のみで解きます。センテンス（主語＋動詞）の形で答えるように心がけてください。他の学習者とペアを組み、読み上げられた質問に対して口頭で答えるとより高度な練習が可能です。ただし、レッスン4及びレッスン12は、問診の練習、レッスン5は英作文の練習になっています。

10　Test
各レッスンの単語が身についているかを確認するため、巻末の Answer Sheet 裏面に単語テストが用意されています。ただし、レッスン4、5、12は問診の練習となっています。

DjD Interview Program（動画付き）
一般の人たちに歯科についてもっと興味を持っていただくことを目指し、日々活動している DjD（The Disc Jockey of Dentistry）によるインタビューコーナーです。現役歯科医師の上村先生、三上先生と歯学部で英語を教えているブライアン先生のお話が聞けます。

巻末 Answer Sheet
切り取り用のミシン目が入っています。授業では、切り取って小テストとして使用することも可能です。

Treatment Procedures

診療にともなう動作

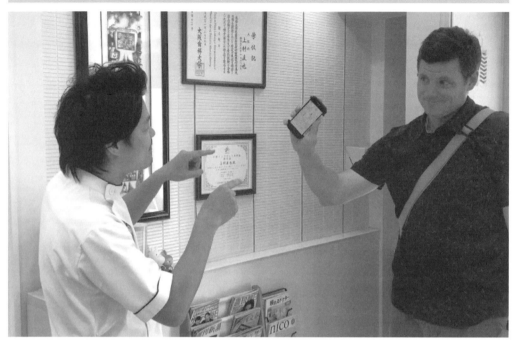

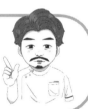

上村先生のワンポイントアドバイス

Patients are under stress during the treatment. Since it can be the cause of fatigue and discomfort, the dentist should try to minimize this stress. Directions to the patient that are well-timed can make the treatment procedures flow very smoothly. As a result, the treatment experience will be successful for both the patient and the dentist.

1 Core Terms
次の語を英語の場合は日本語に、日本語の場合は英語に直しなさい。

1. 開ける

2. 閉じる

3. 噛み合わせる

4. 大きく口を開ける

5. 開けたままにする

6. 楽にする

7. 口をゆすぐ

8. procedure

9. lower

10. raise

11. dental suction

12. treatment

Brian's Pronunciation Practice
動画の音声に続いてリピートしなさい。

1.　open	2.　close	3.　bite down	4.　open wide
5.　keep open	6.　relax	7.　rinse out	8.　procedure
9.　lower	10. raise	11. dental suction	12. treatment

3 Bernie's Pronunciation Tips
患者さんにはクリアな英語を伝える必要があります。
このコーナーでは日本人にとって発音の難しい単語を挙げています。
動画の音声に続いて単語の発音練習をしなさい。

1. right / light　　2. ray / lay　　3. river / liver　　4. rip / lip　　5. row / low

4 Core Phrases
次の英文を和訳しなさい。

1.　I will recline your chair.

2.　Open your mouth, please.

3.　Open wide.

4.　Keep your mouth open.

5.　Please bite down.

6.　You may close your mouth.

7.　Please rinse out your mouth.

8.　I will return your chair.

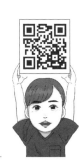

 Quick Response
動画を見て日本語に対する英訳を瞬時に口頭で言いなさい。
瞬発力が大事です！

Risa's Coffee Break

動画を見て、リサ先生の指示に従って英語で言ってみよう。
その後、下の枠に答えを英語で書きなさい。

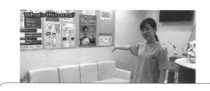

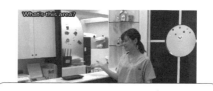

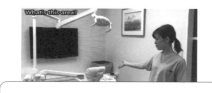

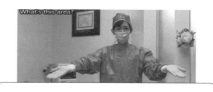

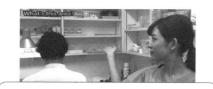

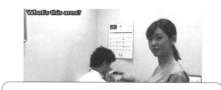

---

7 **Workout**

日常生活と歯科医院での英語表現を確認しよう。

▶ I have...   You have...

日常生活では、「〜を持っている」という意味でよく使うフレーズ。

I have a great idea. すごくいい考えがある。

You have a nice sweater.　いいセーターだね。

歯科医院では、病気の症状や病名を伝える時によく使う。

（患者）　I have a toothache.　私は歯が痛いです。

（患者）　I have a runny nose.　鼻水がでます。

（歯科医）You have canker sores inside your cheeks.　頬の内側に口内炎があります。

次の和文を英作しなさい。

1．あなたは口臭があります。

2．あなたは歯周炎に罹っています。

8 Dialogs
動画を見て次の各空欄を埋めなさい。

Dialog 1 （電話：急な来院）

Dentist: もしもし。

Patient: Hello? I don't have an (   ) ...but can I see you

(   ) (   ) ?

Dentist: What seems to be the problem?

Patient: I have a (   ) (   ) .

Dentist: Oh, no. Please come (   ) (   ) .

May I have your name?

Patient: My name is Peter Parker.

Dentist: OK, Mr. Parker, don't forget to bring your (   )

(   ) .

Patient: Sure. I will be there (   ) (   ) minutes.

Dialog 2 （歯科医院に到着）

Dentist: How is the (   ) outside?

Patient: It's a (   ) day though a bit (   ) .

Dentist: So, how did you get here?

Patient: I walked from the train station.

Dentist: Must have been (   ) finding your way.

Patient: Actually, it was a (   ) .

Dentist: You didn't ask anyone (   ) (   )

(   ) ?

Patient: No need. My smartphone (   ) guides me in English. See?

Dentist: Wow!

9 Listening Comprehension
「8」Dialogs の動画をもう一度見て巻末の Answer Sheet にある問題を解きなさい。

10 Test
巻末の Answer Sheet の裏面にあるテストを受けなさい。

Lesson 2
General Terms
一般的な用語

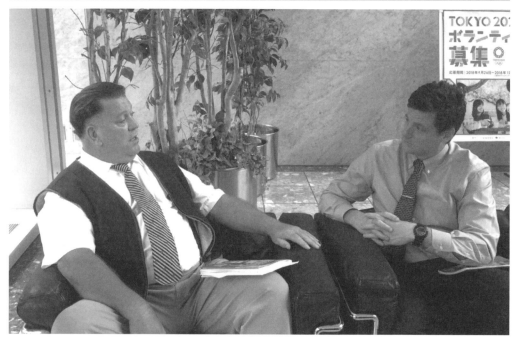

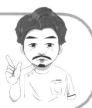
1 Core Terms
次の語を英語の場合は日本語に、日本語の場合は英語に直しなさい。

1. 治療する
2. 歯
3. 虫歯

4. 歯科医院
5. 歯科医師
6. 歯科医学

7. shed
8. erupt
9. primary teeth

10. permanent teeth
11. stains

2 Brian's Pronunciation Practice
動画の音声に続いてリピートしなさい。

1.　treat	2.　tooth	3.　cavity
4.　dental clinic	5.　dentist	6.　Dentistry
7.　shed	8.　erupt	9.　primary teeth
10. permanent teeth	11. stains	

3 Bernie's Pronunciation Tips
患者さんにはクリアな英語を伝える必要があります。
このコーナーでは日本人にとって発音の難しい単語を挙げています。
動画の音声に続いて単語の発音練習をしなさい。

1. tooth　　2. health　　3. mouth　　4. forth　　5. throbbing

4 Core Phrases
次の英文を和訳しなさい。

1.　A dental clinic is where you get your teeth treated.

2.　The hygienist assisted the dentist during the checkup.

3.　This treatment requires several visits.

4.　The primary teeth start to erupt from about 6 months of age.

5.　Baby teeth shed at various times during childhood.

6.　Permanent teeth begin erupting at 6 years of age.

7.　Dental students study Dentistry at dental school.

5 Quick Response
動画を見て日本語に対する英訳を瞬時に
口頭で言いなさい。瞬発力が大事です！

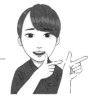

6 Risa's Coffee Break
動画を見て、リサ先生の指示に従って英語で言ってみよう。
その後、下の枠に答えを英語で書きなさい。

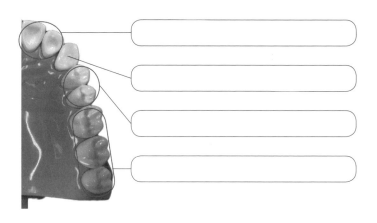

7 Workout
次の各空欄を埋めなさい。

一般用語（lay term）＝ 専門用語（technical term）

1.　(　　　　　　　　)(　　　　　　　　　　) ＝ anterior teeth
2.　　　　　tarta　　　　　　　　＝ (　　　　　　　　)
3.　　　　　cavity　　　　　　　　＝ (　　　　　　　　)
4.　(　　　　　　　　)(　　　　　　　　　　) ＝ primary teeth
5.　　　　adult teeth　　　　　　＝ (　　　　　)(　　　　　)
6.　　　　(　　　　　　　　　) ＝ gingiva
7.　　　　bite（名詞）　　　　　　＝ (　　　　　　　　)
8.　(　　　　　　　)(　　　　　　　) ＝ posterior teeth
9.　　　　braces　　　　　　　　＝ (　　　　　)(　　　　　)
10. (　　　　　　)(　　　　　　　) ＝ third molar

7

8 Dialogs
動画を見て次の各空欄を埋めなさい。

Dialog 1（友人の歯が気になって…。）

Peter:　Bill, when was the last time you had a
　　　　(　　　　　　　) (　　　　　　　　　　) the dentist?

Bill:　　A few years back when I was in the United States. Why?

Peter:　Well, I noticed you have (　　　　　　　) (　　　　　　　　　)
　　　　(　　　　　　　) (　　　　　　　　　) on the front of your teeth.

Bill:　　Yeah, I think I'm...maybe I am drinking too much (　　　　　　　　)
　　　　(　　　　　　　) (　　　　　　　　　) . Is it that bad?

Peter:　It's pretty bad recently. Why don't you (　　　　　　　　)
　　　　my (　　　　　　　) ?
　　　　He is very skilled and the (　　　　　　　　) does a wonderful job.

Bill:　　Can they speak English?

Peter:　They can.

Bill:　　Really? Okay, great. So, tell me where are they?

Peter:　Here, I can show you.

Dialog 2（英語が話せる歯科医師いる？）

Bill:　　Have you been to a (　　　　　　　　) (　　　　　　　　　) in Japan?

Peter:　Yes, I visit (　　　　　　　) (　　　　　　　　) (　　　　　　　　　)
　　　　(　　　　　　　) .

Bill:　　Is the dentist skilled and easy to (　　　　　　　　) (　　　　　　　　) ?

Peter:　Yes, and he speaks English well.

Bill:　　Sounds nice. That means you can ask about (　　　　　　　　) ,
　　　　(　　　　　　　) , and (　　　　　　　) ?

Peter:　Yes, that's why I am a (　　　　　　　　) (　　　　　　　　　) .

9 Listening Comprehension
「8」Dialogsの動画をもう一度見て巻末のAnswer Sheetにある問題を解きなさい。

10 Test
巻末の Answer Sheet の裏面にあるテストを受けなさい。

Parts of the Mouth

各部の名称

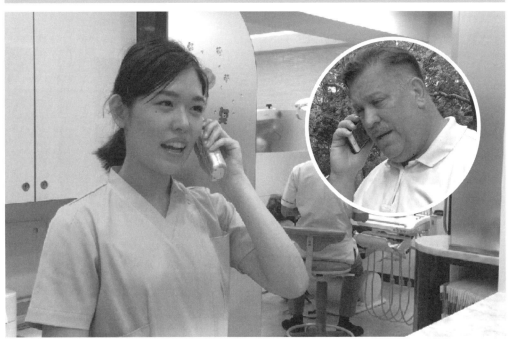

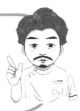

上村先生のワンポイントアドバイス

As a student, I studied English by memorizing words and phrases by sight. That is, I would prepare flash cards with English on one side and Japanese on the other. I would look at the words and try to immediately come up with the translation. In reality, foreign patients do not show you flash cards when speaking English. That is why improving your listening comprehension is important.

1 Core Terms
次の語を英語の場合は日本語に、日本語の場合は英語に直しなさい。

1. 舌	2. 唇	3. 頬	4. 上顎
5. 下顎	6. membrane	7. joint	8. gums
9. root	10. crown	11. canines	12. molars
13. premolars	14. incisors	15. saliva	

2 **Brian's Pronunciation Practice**
動画の音声に続いてリピートしなさい。

1. tongue	2. lip(s)	3. cheek(s)	4. upper jaw
5. lower jaw	6. membrane	7. joint	8. gums
9. root	10. crown	11. canines	12. molars
13. premolars	14. incisors	15. saliva	

3 **Bernie's Pronunciation Tips**
患者さんにはクリアな英語を伝える必要があります。
このコーナーでは日本人にとって発音の難しい単語を挙げています。
動画の音声に続いて単語の発音練習をしなさい。

1. saliva   2. alignment   3. side   4. grind   5. incisors

4 **Core Phrases**
次の英文を和訳しなさい。

1. Canines tear food.

2. Molars grind food during chewing.

3. Incisors cut food into small pieces.

4. Premolars tear and crush food.

5. The gums are the tissue that surrounds the base of the teeth.

6. Teeth can be divided into the crown and the root.

5 **Quick Response**
動画を見て日本語に対する英訳を瞬時に口頭で言いなさい。
瞬発力が大事です！

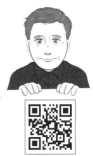

10

Risa's Coffee Break
動画を見て、ブライアン先生と一緒に発音しなさい。

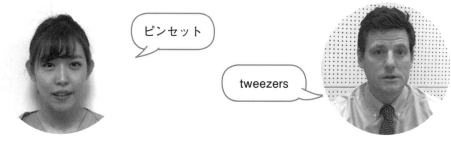

ピンセット

tweezers

Risa

Brian

 Workout
次の各定義が示している英語を書きなさい。
その後、動画を見てすぐに答えられるように練習しなさい。

1. The soft muscular organ used for such functions as tasting, eating, and speaking

2. The two fleshy parts that form the opening of the mouth

3. The fleshy wall of the mouth on either side of the face

4. The tissue that surrounds the roots of the teeth

5. The two bone structures that form the framework of the mouth

6. The fluid secreted in the mouth from glands for lubricating, chewing, and swallowing

 Dialogs
動画を見て次の各空欄を埋めなさい。

Dialog 1（電話：緊急）

Patient: Hello. May I talk to the dentist? (　　　　　　) (　　　　　　)
(　　　　　　) .

Dentist: Hello. What happened?

Patient: I was eating a sticky pecan pie and my crown (　　　　　　)
(　　　　　　) .

11

Dentist: Did you (　　　　　　　　) it?

Patient: Fortunately not. I have it here in my hand.

Dentist: You must come to the clinic (　　　　　　) (　　　　　　).

Patient: But I can't. I am on vacation. Is it o.k. if I (　　　　　　)

(　　　　　　) (　　　　　　) (　　　　　　)

with some adhesive like superglue?

Dentist: No! Don't do anything like that.

Patient: Then I will see you when I return (　　　　　　) (　　　　　　)

(　　　　　　) (　　　　　　).

In the meantime what should I do?

Dentist: (　　　　　　) (　　　　　　) (　　　　　　) keep it clean

by brushing softly. O.K.? Your tooth might be (　　　　　　)

(　　　　　　) hot or cold drinks and food.

Patient: Gotcha. Thanks, doc.

[注] pecan pie ＝ ペカンナッツとコーンシロップで作る甘いパイ

Dialog 2（虫歯の治療で来たけど…。）

Dentist: Hello, Peter.

Patient: Hello, Doctor. You are going to treat my cavity today, right?

Dentist: That's correct. (　　　　　　) (　　　　　　)?

Patient: Well, something hurts on the inside of my (　　　　　　)

(　　　　　　).

Dentist: Let's take a look…Oh, you have a large (　　　　　　)

(　　　　　　).

Patient: It hurts pretty bad. Can we (　　　　　　) treatment?

Dentist: Yes. I think that's a good idea. I will (　　　　　　) the sore and

(　　　　　　) some steroids.

Patient: OK.

9 Listening Comprehension

「8」Dialogs の動画をもう一度見て巻末の Answer Sheet にある問題を解きなさい。

10 Test

巻末の Answer Sheet の裏面にあるテストを受けなさい。

DjD interview program

本日のゲスト ☛ Dr. Naoya Uemura

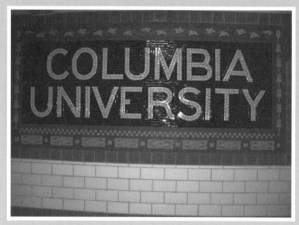

116th Street Station

Dr. Uemura spent time at Columbia University in New York City. His specialty is implant treatment.

DjD did research at Columbia University. There is a great difference in funding between Japan and the U.S.

The key to improving your English is to go abroad. All you need is some confidence and some money.

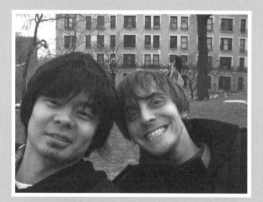

Dr. Uemura and his friend

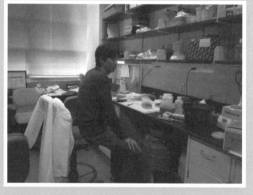

DjD researching

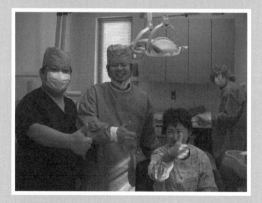

At the Clinic

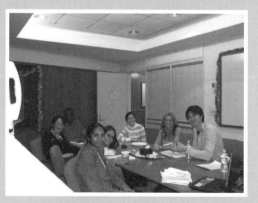

DjD with fellow researchers

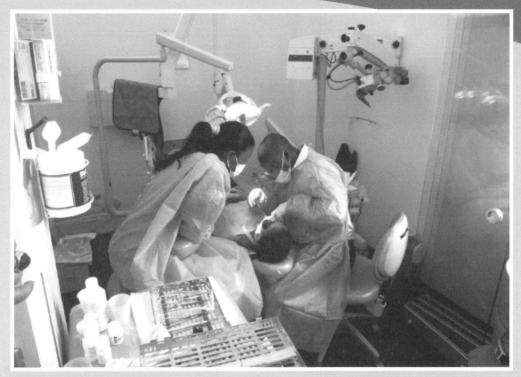
Treatment at the university hospital

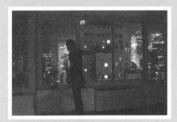
DjD's apartment on 33rd St.

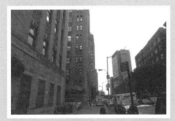
New York Presbyterian Hospital

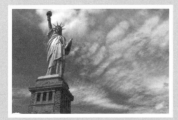
The Statue of Liberty

New Yorkers in the subway wear hooded sweatshirts and look into the tunnel waiting for the next train.

Dr. Uemura jogged and played tennis in Central Park. DjD jogged along the Hudson River.

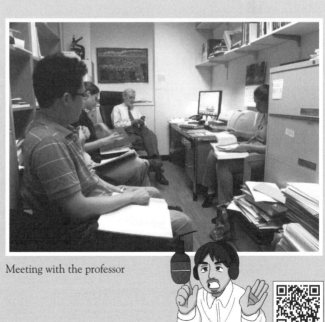
Meeting with the professor

Lesson 4

Interview
問診に必要な用語

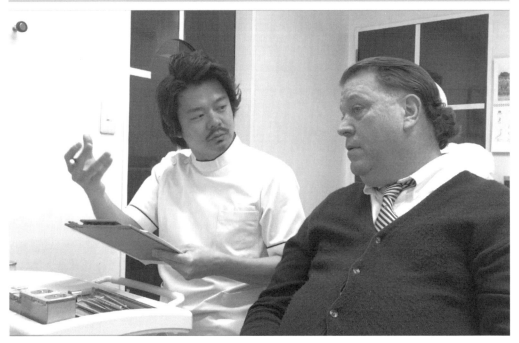

上村先生のワンポイントアドバイス

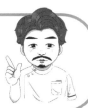

As a new dentist on the job, you try so hard and sometimes end up doing "too much" for the patient. On the other hand, time constraints can lead to doing "too little." Whatever treatment you do, I think accuracy and consistency is most important.

1 Core Terms
次の語を英語の場合は日本語に、日本語の場合は英語に直しなさい。

1. 患者への問診　　2. 痛む（h）　　3. 痛む（a）　　4. 血

5. 出血する　　6. dull pain　　7. sharp pain　　8. throbbing pain

9. sensitive to ～　　10. numb　　11. nerve　　12. feel loose

13. discomfort　　14. swollen gums　　15. tooth extraction

2 Brian's Pronunciation Practice
動画の音声に続いてリピートしなさい。

1. patient interview 2. hurt 3. ache 4. blood
5. bleed 6. dull pain 7. sharp pain 8. throbbing pain
9. sensitive to 10. numb 11. nerve 12. feel loose
13. discomfort 14. swollen gums 15. tooth extraction

3 Bernie's Pronunciation Tips
患者さんにはクリアな英語を伝える必要があります。
このコーナーでは日本人にとって発音の難しい単語を挙げています。
動画の音声に続いて単語の発音練習をしなさい。

1. hurt 2. curve 3. surface 4. nerve 5. serve

4 Core Phrases
次の英文を和訳しなさい。

1. What seems to be the problem?

2. Is this your first visit to this clinic?

3. Where is the pain?

4. When did the pain start?

5. What kind of pain is it?

6. Have you ever had a tooth extraction?

7. Did you experience any problems then?

5 Quick Response
動画を見て日本語に対する英訳を瞬時に口頭で
言いなさい。瞬発力が大事です！

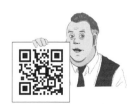

6 Risa's Coffee Break

動画を見て、リサ先生の指示に従って英語で言ってみよう。

その後、下の枠に答えを英語で書きなさい。

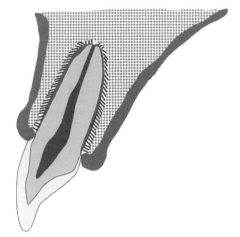

1.

2.

3.

4.

5.

6.

7.

---

7 Workout

日常生活と歯科医院での英語表現を確認しよう。

▶ There is...

日常生活では、「〜がある」という意味でよく使うフレーズ。

There is a new café on the corner.　角に新しいカフェがある。

There is not any gas in the tank.　タンクにはガソリンはない。

There are some questions I'd like to ask.　聞きたい質問がいくつかあります。

歯科医院では、

患者のお口の状態を伝える（診断を伝える）時に使う。

There is a canker sore on the tip of your tongue.　舌尖に口内炎が出来ています。

主語をYouにして "You have..." でも同じ意味となる。

You have a canker sore on the tip of your tongue.

次の和文を英作しなさい。

1．前歯にひどい着色があります。

2．う蝕の可能性があります。

8 Dialogs
動画を見て次の各空欄を埋めなさい。

Dialog 1 （問診：どうなさいましたか？）

Dentist: What seems to be the problem?

Patient: My tooth aches especially when I eat (　　　　　　　)
(　　　　　　　).

Dentist: Is this your first visit to this clinic?

Patient: Yes, it is.

Dentist: Where is the pain?

Patient: It seems to be in one of my (　　　　　　　) (　　　　　　　)
(　　　　　　　). I think it is the (　　　　　　　)
(　　　　　　　) from the back.

Dentist: When did the pain start?

Patient: About last week when I was (　　　　　　　) on some nuts.

Dialog 2 （問診：痛みについて）

Dentist: What kind of pain is it?

Patient: It is a (　　　　　　　) (　　　　　　　) except when I chew on it.
Then, it's a (　　　　　　　) (　　　　　　　).

Dentist: Have you ever had a tooth extraction?

Patient: Extraction?

Dentist: Removed.

Patient: Yes, I had a (　　　　　　　) (　　　　　　　) taken out.

Dentist: Did you experience any problems then?

Patient: No.

9 Practice
動画（Case1）を見て、巻末のAnswer Sheetにバーニー先生の質問文を予測して書きなさい。裏面（Case2）でブライアン先生に合わせて質問文を言いなさい。

10 Role Playing
巻末のAnswer Sheetを使ってロールプレイングで問診の練習をしなさい。

Lesson 5
Interview 2
問診に必要な用語

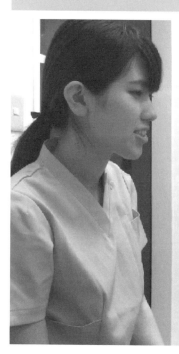
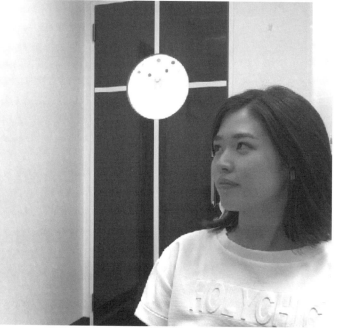

上村先生のワンポイントアドバイス

It is important to be extra sure that the patients do not have any allergies. Sometimes, they can be the cause of unexpected troubles. Allergic reactions to certain medicines can in some cases be life threatening. Metals can also cause allergy.

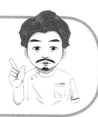

1 **Core Terms**
次の語を英語の場合は日本語に、日本語の場合は英語に直しなさい。

1. 血圧	2. アレルギー	3. 健康保険
4. side effect	5. medication	6. anesthetic
7. diabetes	8. pregnant	9. buildup
10. symptom	11. hay fever	12. tartar

2 Brian's Pronunciation Practice
動画の音声に続いてリピートしなさい。

1. blood pressure
2. allergy
3. health insurance
4. side effect
5. medication
6. anesthetic
7. diabetes
8. pregnant
9. buildup
10. symptom
11. hay fever
12. tartar

3 Bernie's Pronunciation Tips
患者さんにはクリアな英語を伝える必要があります。
このコーナーでは日本人にとって発音の難しい単語を挙げています。
動画の音声に続いて単語の発音練習をしなさい。

1. allergy　2. anesthetic　3. apple　4. cavity　5. relax

4 Core Phrases
次の英文を和訳しなさい。

1. Do you have any allergies?

2. Have you experienced any side effects from medication?

3. Are you pregnant?

4. Is there anything else that bothers you?

5. Do you have health insurance?

6. Any other requests or concerns?

5 Quick Response
動画を見て日本語に対する英訳を瞬時に口頭で言いなさい。
瞬発力が大事です！

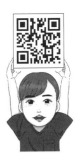

Risa's Coffee Break
動画を見て、ブライアン先生と一緒に発音しなさい。

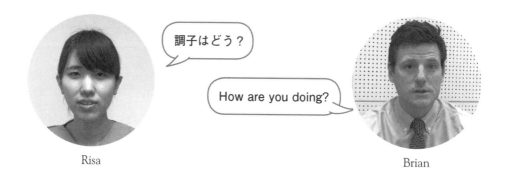

調子はどう？

How are you doing?

Risa

Brian

 Workout
次の各質問に対して（　　）内の単語を使って
英語で答えを書きなさい。
その後、ペアになって口頭で練習しなさい。

1. Q : What are you allergic to? あなたは何に対してアレルギーを持っていますか。

   A : I am ....

   たまご：

   ねこ：

   麻酔：

2. Q : Do you have any allergies? アレルギーはありますか。

   A : I have ....

   食べ物：

   花粉：

   金属：

3. Q : What are your symptoms? 症状は何ですか。

   A : I have ....

   かゆみ：

   発熱：

   胃の痛み：

   発疹：

Dialogs
動画を見て次の各空欄を埋めなさい。

Dialog 1 （問診：アレルギー）

Dentist: Do you have any allergies?

Patient: I have (　　　　　　　) (　　　　　　　　　), otherwise no.

Dentist: Have you experienced any side effects from medication?

Patient: No, I haven't.

Dentist: Are you pregnant?

Patient: Yes, I am (　　　　　　) (　　　　　　) (　　　　　　).

Dialog 2 （問診：他に何か？）

Dentist: Is there anything else that bothers you?

Patient: No, only this (　　　　　　).

Dentist: Do you prefer treatment for just this problem?
　　　　Or, are there any other problems?

Patient: It has been a while since I had my (　　　　　) (　　　　　).
　　　　Could you check for any (　　　　　　)?

Dentist: Do you have health insurance?

Patient: Yes, I am (　　　　　　).

9 **Writing Practice**
巻末のAnswer Sheetの表面を使って問診の英文を書きなさい。

 Interview and Role Playing
巻末のAnswer Sheetの裏面を使って患者に対する質問事項を言いなさい。

Lesson 6

Examination

診察

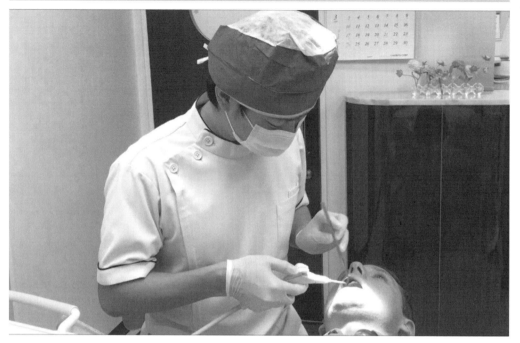

上村先生のワンポイントアドバイス

What should you look for during oral examinations? Certainly, the dentist must be able to detect any abnormalities in the patient's oral region. Being able to distinguish between normal and abnormal requires training and years of experience.

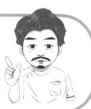

1 Core Terms
次の語を英語の場合は日本語に、日本語の場合は英語に直しなさい。

1. レントゲン	2. 吹きつける	3. 鏡	4. ピンセット
5. 予約 (a)	6. 細菌	7. examination	8. alignment
9. sensitivity	10. periodontal pocket	11. depth	12. plaque
13. explorer	14. inter-dental brush		

2

Brian's Pronunciation Practice
動画の音声に続いてリピートしなさい。

1. x–ray	2. blow	3. mirror	4. tweezers
5. appointment	6. bacteria	7. examination	8. alignment
9. sensitivity	10. periodontal pocket	11. depth	12. plaque
13. explorer	14. inter-dental brush		

 3

Bernie's Pronunciation Tips
患者さんにはクリアな英語を伝える必要があります。
このコーナーでは日本人にとって発音の難しい単語を挙げています。
動画の音声に続いて単語の発音練習をしなさい。

1. x–ray　　2. exile　　3. xylitol　　4. anxiety　　5. luxury
※同じ "x" でも発音が異なります。

 4

Core Phrases
次の英文を和訳しなさい。

1. I am going to examine your teeth alignment.

2. I'm going to blow air on your teeth.

3. I am going to examine your periodontal pocket.

4. I will check your gums for bleeding.

5. I will take an x–ray of your cavity.

 5

Quick Response
動画を見て日本語に対する英訳を瞬時に口頭で言いなさい。
瞬発力が大事です！

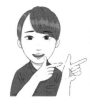

Risa's Coffee Break
動画を見て、ブライアン先生と一緒に発音しなさい。

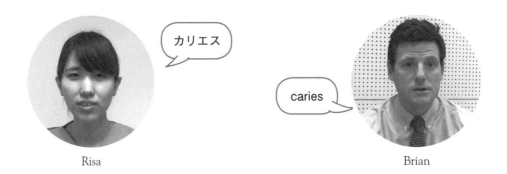

カリエス

caries

Risa

Brian

7 Workout
日常生活と歯科医院での英語表現を確認しよう。

▶ I will...　　I am going to...

日常生活では、

I will go to New York City.

I am going to New York City.

両方とも「私はニューヨークへ行きます」と訳せます。しかし、ニュアンスに若干の違いがあります。"Will" を使った場合は、ニューヨークへ行こうという本人の強い意志を表現しています。それに対して、"am going to" はニューヨークへ行くことになっているという事実を表現している。

歯科医院では、

治療の時に何も言わずに麻酔を注射する歯科医師はいません。必ず、次のステップを説明しながら、"I will inject anesthetic to your gums"（これから歯茎に麻酔を注射します）という声掛けをします。日常会話のように細かいニュアンスを気にする必要はないため "will" と "am going to" の両方を使います。大事なのは必ず次のステップを伝えることです。

次の和文を英作しなさい。

1．歯と歯茎の間の溝の深さを測ります。

2．歯にフッ化物を塗布します。

8 Dialogs
動画を見て次の各空欄を埋めなさい。

Dialog 1 （電話：予約）

Dentist:　　Hello?

Bill Smith:　Hello, I would like to (　　　　　) (　　　　　)
　　　　　　(　　　　　).

Dentist:　　What seems to be the problem?

Bill Smith:　My tooth hurts when I (　　　　　) (　　　　　)
　　　　　　(　　　　　).

Dentist:　　OK, how about tomorrow morning?

Bill Smith:　I (　　　　　) (　　　　　) (　　　　　) in the
　　　　　　morning. (　　　　　) (　　　　　) after 4 pm?

Dentist:　　I can fit you in at 6:30.

Bill Smith:　OK.

Dentist:　　(　　　　　) (　　　　　) (　　　　　)
　　　　　　(　　　　　) (　　　　　)?

Bill Smith:　My name is Bill Smith.

Dentist:　　All right. See you at 6:30 tomorrow evening, Mr. Smith.

Dialog 2 （プラークって何？）

Dentist: You have (　　　　　) (　　　　　) between your teeth.

Patient: What is plaque?

Dentist: It is a (　　　　　) (　　　　　) that contains bacteria.

Patient: Is it harmful?

Dentist: It may eventually lead to (　　　　　) and (　　　　　)
　　　　　(　　　　　).

Patient: Do you think using dental floss would be effective?

Dentist: Absolutely. You may also use an (　　　　　) (　　　　　).

9 Listening Comprehension
「8」Dialogs の動画をもう一度見て巻末の Answer Sheet にある問題を
解きなさい。

10 Test
巻末の Answer Sheet の裏面にあるテストを受けなさい。

DjD interview program

本日のゲスト ☛ Dr. Yu Mikami

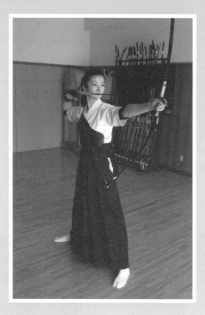

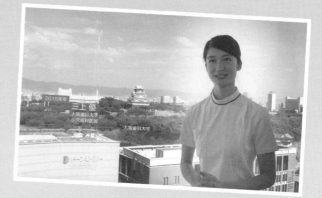

Yu practiced Japanese Archery in the university club. She learned the importance of manners and respecting seniority.

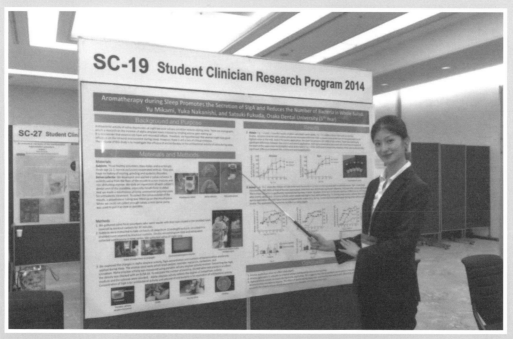

Yu started research on the effect of aromas from her second year. She stayed up all night collecting saliva samples.

Yu was one of the finalists of the Miss Nippon 2017 contest

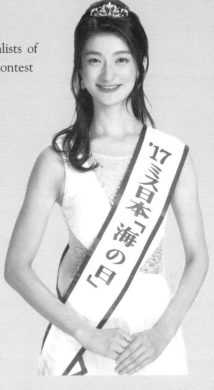

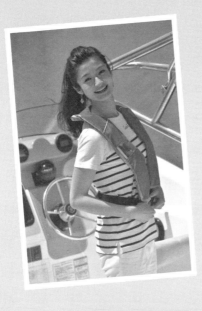

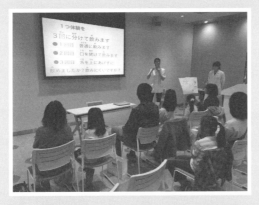

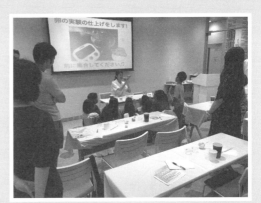

Yu has been interested in promoting oral health. As a specialist in pediatric dentistry, she participates in events for children where they learn how to brush properly and even make their own toothpaste!

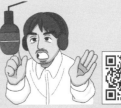

Diagnosis
診断

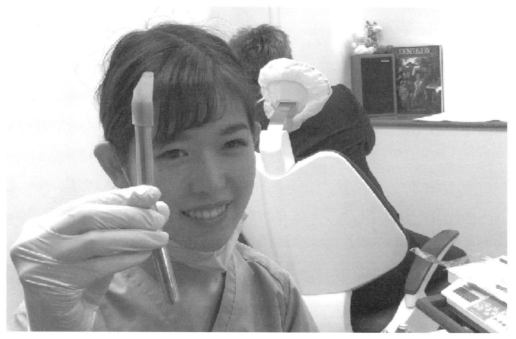

上村先生のワンポイントアドバイス

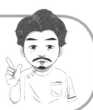

The ability to reach an accurate diagnosis of the patient's condition is one of the qualities required to become a good dentist. Like oral examinations, this can only be obtained through years of training and years of experience.

1 Core Terms
次の語を英語の場合は日本語に、日本語の場合は英語に直しなさい。

1. 診断

2. 細菌感染

3. 口腔乾燥症

4. 口臭

5. 病気

6. tooth decay

7. ill–fitting denture

8. inflammation

9. demineralization

10. periodontitis

11. receding gums

12. pus

Brian's Pronunciation Practice
動画の音声に続いてリピートしなさい。

1. diagnosis
2. bacterial infection
3. dry mouth
4. bad breath
5. disease
6. tooth decay
7. ill-fitting denture
8. inflammation
9. demineralization
10. periodontitis
11. receding gums
12. pus

 Bernie's Pronunciation Tips
患者さんにはクリアな英語を伝える必要があります。
このコーナーでは日本人にとって発音の難しい単語を挙げています。
動画の音声に続いて単語の発音練習をしなさい。

1. ill　2. fitting　3. inflammation　4. disease　5. infection

4　Core Phrases
次の英文を和訳しなさい。

1. There is a hole in the tooth caused by decay.

2. There is mineral loss from the teeth.

3. You drink too much coffee and wine.

4. You have brushed too hard over a long period of time.

5. Maybe you eat a lot of strong smelling food.

6. What happens if gum disease is left untreated?

7. There is a reduction of saliva due to medication.

 Quick Response
動画を見て日本語に対する英訳を瞬時に口頭で言いなさい。
瞬発力が大事です！

6 Risa's Coffee Break

動画を見て、リサ先生の指示に従って英語で言ってみよう。
その後、下の枠に答えを英語で書きなさい。

①

②

③

④

⑤

7 Workout

下記の文と一致する病名あるいは症状を選びなさい。
その後、動画を見て口頭で病名あるいは症状を回答できるように練習しましょう。

1. There is a hole in the tooth caused by decay.
2. There is mineral loss from the teeth.
3. You drink too much coffee and wine.
4. You have brushed too hard over a long period of time.
5. You eat a lot of strong smelling food.
6. Gum disease is left untreated.
7. There is a reduction of saliva due to medication.

a. extrinsic stain   b. periodontitis   c. cavity / caries   d. bad breath
e. demineralization   f. receding gums   g. dry mouth

8 Dialogs

動画を見て次の各空欄を埋めなさい。

Dialog 1（虫歯のようですね。）

Patient: I've been having some pain in my (　　　　　) (　　　　　)
(　　　　　) .

Dentist: Let me (　　　　　) (　　　　　) (　　　　　)
(　　　　　) them and see what is wrong.

Patient: Oooh! The second one from the back is (　　　　　) .

Dentist: You either have (　　　　　) (　　　　　) or some
hyper–sensitivity. Open wide.

Patient: Could it be a cavity?

Dentist: It sure is...and quite deep, too.

Dialog 2（奥歯が痛みますが…。）

Patient: The area surrounding my lower back tooth (　　　　　)
(　　　　　) .

Dentist: Let's see. Open wide.

Patient: So, what's wrong?

Dentist: The (　　　　　) of your rear teeth are (　　　　　) .
Let's (　　　　　) (　　　　　) (　　　　　) and
check.

Patient: How bad is it?

Dentist: As you can see here, you have pus formation and the wisdom tooth is
(　　　　　) . It is called an (　　　　　)
(　　　　　) .

［注］tender ＝ 圧痛のある　　pus formation ＝ 化膿

9 Listening Comprehension

動画をもう一度見て巻末の Answer Sheet にある問題を解きなさい。

10 Test

巻末の Answer Sheet の裏面にあるテストを受けなさい。

Lesson 8

Treatment Procedures 2
診療にともなう動作

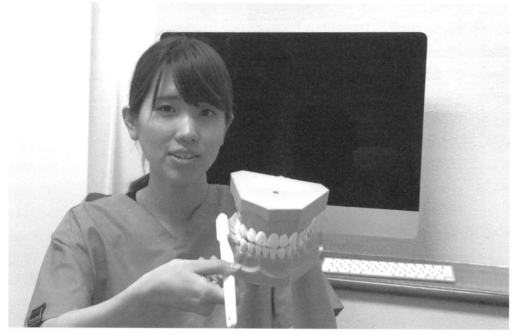

上村先生のワンポイントアドバイス

Even the slightest bumps or edges on the tooth surface can be the cause of much discomfort. The treatment itself may have been successful with the removal of the decayed part of the tooth. However, no treatment can be considered complete without the finishing touches.

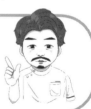

1 Core Terms
次の語を英語の場合は日本語に、日本語の場合は英語に直しなさい。

1. 前後	2. 左右	3. なぞる (r)
4. 荒い	5. gargle	6. clench
7. grind	8. bumps or edges	9. chip
10. composite resin	11. bond（動詞）	12. polish

2 Brian's Pronunciation Practice
動画の音声に続いてリピートしなさい。

1. back and forth
2. sideways
3. run
4. rough
5. gargle
6. clench
7. grind
8. bumps or edges
9. chip
10. composite resin
11. bond（動詞）
12. polish

3 Bernie's Pronunciation Tips
患者さんにはクリアな英語を伝える必要があります。
このコーナーでは日本人にとって発音の難しい単語を挙げています。
動画の音声に続いて単語の発音練習をしなさい。

1. clench　　2. clean　　3. clinic　　4. cleanse　　5. close

4 Core Phrases
次の英文を和訳しなさい。

1. Grind your teeth a little.

2. It may hurt a little.

3. Do you feel pain?

4. Run your tongue along it.

5. Do you feel any bumps or edges?

5 Quick Response
動画を見て日本語に対する英訳を瞬時に口頭で言いなさい。
瞬発力が大事です！

6 Risa's Coffee Break
動画を見て、バーニー先生と一緒に歯磨き指導を英語で言ってみよう。

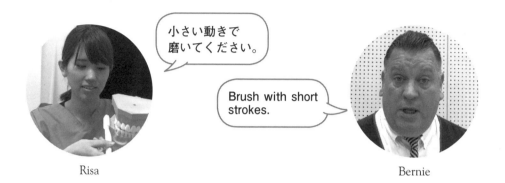

小さい動きで
磨いてください。

Brush with short
strokes.

Risa

Bernie

---

7 Workout
日常生活と歯科医院での英語表現を確認しよう。

▶ How about...?

日常会話では、
相手を誘うときによく使うフレーズです。
例えば、How about some coffee?　コーヒーでもどう？

歯科医院では、
患者が使うとき（相手の意見や考えを求めて）
Patient:　How about whitening treatment?
　　　　　ホワイトニング治療をしたらいいでしょうか。
Dentist:　I think it would be effective.　効果があると思いますよ。

歯科医師が使うとき（提案）
Dentist:　How about orthodontic treatment?　歯科矯正をされてはいかがですか。
Patient:　What kind of treatment is it?　それはどのような治療ですか。

次の和文を英作しなさい。
1. 来週の水曜日の午後はいかがでしょうか。

2. セラミッククラウンにされたらいかがでしょうか。見た目が自然です。

8 **Dialogs**
動画を見て次の各空欄を埋めなさい。

Dialog 1（アクシデント）

Dentist:　What's wrong?

Patient:　I (　　　　　　　　) and (　　　　　　　　　) on my face.

Dentist:　Oh, that's awful.

Patient:　I think I (　　　　　　　　) (　　　　　　　　) (　　　　　　　　).

Dentist:　Let me take a look...seems like you chipped your (　　　　　　　　)
　　　　　(　　　　　　　　).

Patient:　What can be done about it?

Dentist:　Since you chipped off only a small piece, I will bond the tooth using
　　　　　(　　　　　　　　) (　　　　　　　　) (　　　　　　　　)
　　　　　(　　　　　　　　).

Patient: How long will it take?

Dentist: I can do it right now. It won't take long.

［注］trip ＝つまずく

Dialog 2（仕上げに…。）

Dentist: Try grinding your teeth (　　　　　　　　) and (　　　　　　　　) and
　　　　　(　　　　　　　　). How does it feel?

Patient: It fits well.

Dentist: Could you (　　　　　　　　) (　　　　　　　　) (　　　　　　　　)
　　　　　around the filling?

Patient: Yes.

Dentist: Do you feel any (　　　　　　　　) or (　　　　　　　　)?

Patient: The surface feels a little rough on my tongue.

Dentist: O.K. I will (　　　　　　　　) (　　　　　　　　) the edge. Open wide.
　　　　　So, how does it feel now?

Patient: Very smooth. Much more comfortable.

Dentist: Please rinse out your mouth.

9 **Listing Comprehension**
「8」Dialogsの動画をもう一度見て巻末のAnswer Sheetにある問題を解きなさい。

10 **Test**
巻末のAnswer Sheetの裏面にあるテストを受けなさい。

Lesson 9
Treating Cavities
虫歯

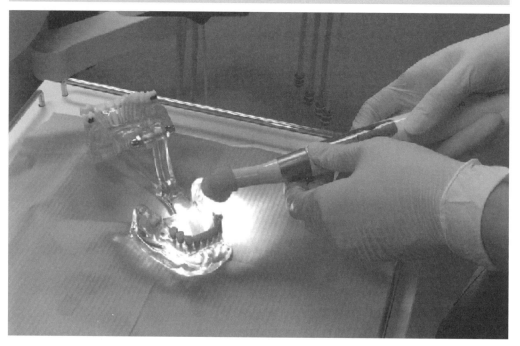

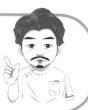

上村先生のワンポイントアドバイス

For patients, it can be quite shocking when they are diagnosed as having a cavity. It is the dentist's role to express consideration towards the patient's feelings and encourage them to start treatment.

1 Core Terms
次の語を英語の場合は日本語に、日本語の場合は英語に直しなさい。

1. 深い

2. 削る

3. 取り除く

4. 消毒する

5. 詰める

6. 塗る／打つ／照射する

7. 硬くする

8. caries

9. temporary filling

10. permanent filling

11. root canal

12. debris

13. fracture

14. cleanse

2 Brian's Pronunciation Practice
動画の音声に続いてリピートしなさい。

1. deep
2. drill
3. remove
4. disinfect
5. fill
6. apply
7. harden
8. caries
9. temporary filling
10. permanent filling
11. root canal
12. debris
13. fracture
14. cleanse

3 Bernie's Pronunciation Tips
患者さんにはクリアな英語を伝える必要があります。
このコーナーでは日本人にとって発音の難しい単語を挙げています。
動画の音声に続いて単語の発音練習をしなさい。

1. apply   2. deny   3. rely   4. satisfy   5. ally

4 Core Phrases
次の英文を和訳しなさい。

1. I am going to apply local anesthetic to the gums.

2. I will remove the decayed parts of the tooth.

3. I will disinfect the area.

4. I will use a tooth colored filling and apply light to it.

5. I will trim off the rough edges and polish it.

5 Quick Response
動画を見て日本語に対する英訳を瞬時に口頭で言いなさい。
瞬発力が大事です！

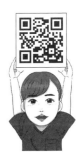

Risa's Coffee Break

動画を見て、リサ先生の指示に従って英語で言ってみよう。

その後、下の枠に答えを英語で書きなさい。

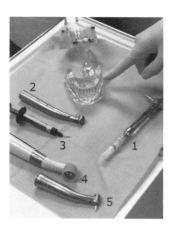

1.

2.

3.

4.

5.

 Workout

次の各質問はどの科の先生に尋ねますか。答えを選びなさい。

その後、動画を見て口頭で科目名を回答できるようにしましょう。

1. You want to know about the structure of the oral region.
2. You want to know about cell metabolism.
3. You want to know whether fluoride is effective or not.
4. You want to know how saliva is secreted.
5. You want to know the different properties of metals.
6. You want to know about Streptococcus mutans.
7. You want to know how drugs are effective.
8. You want to know the mechanism of oral diseases.

ア Pharmacology	イ Anatomy	ウ Bacteriology	エ Biochemistry
オ Pathology	カ Physiology	キ Oral Health	ク Dental Materials

 Dialogs

動画を見て次の各空欄を埋めなさい。

Dialog 1（歯がすごく痛むんだ…。）

Dentist: What's wrong?

Patient: My (　　　　) (　　　　) (　　　　)
　　　　hurts...on the right side.

Dentist: Since when?

Patient: It started a few days ago. But now I (　　　　) (　　　　)
　　　　(　　　　).

Dentist: Let's see. Open wide. You have a big cavity in your (　　　　)
　　　　(　　　　) (　　　　).
　　　　Let's take an x-ray for more detail.

Dentist: As this image on the monitor shows, the cavity is quite deep and the
　　　　(　　　　) (　　　　) (　　　　) (　　　　).

Patient: Oh no. What needs to be done?

Dentist: I suggest we do (　　　　) (　　　　) (　　　　).

Patient: Starting now?

Dentist: Today, I will put a (　　　　) (　　　　) in to stop the
　　　　pain. We will start the treatment in a couple of days.

Dialog 2（治療手順の説明）

Dentist: Look at the x-ray. The discolored area shows (　　　　)
　　　　(　　　　) (　　　　) (　　　　).

Patient: Is it serious?

Dentist: I'm afraid so. It has (　　　　) (　　　　)
　　　　(　　　　). You will need root canal treatment.

Patient: What are you going to do?

Dentist: I will (　　　　) (　　　　) the decayed area.
　　　　Then I will disinfect the root canal. Finally, I will fill the tooth and
　　　　(　　　　) it with a metal crown.

Patient: Will it be painful?

Dentist: Don't worry. There will be (　　　　) (　　　　) than now.

Patient: How many visits will it take?

Dentist: I would say about 5 or 6 visits.

9 Listening Comprehension
「8」Dialogsの動画をもう一度見て巻末のAnswer Sheetにある問題を解きなさい。

10 Test
巻末のAnswer Sheetの裏面にあるテストを受けなさい。

DjD interview program

本日のゲスト ☛ Mr. Brian Bachman

Boston is about the same size as Kyoto. It is famous for lobsters and other delicious food. The Patriots who have just won the Super Bowl and the Red Sox are popular local teams.

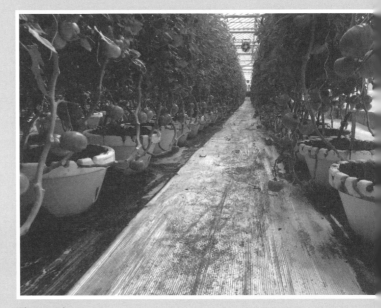
The greenhouse

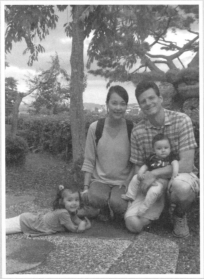
Brian and his family

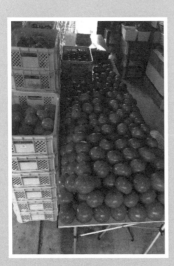
Ripe tomatoes

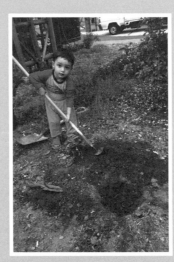
A little farmer

Brian is a farmer in Kyoto. There are two greenhouses with 4000 tomato plants including mini-tomatoes and beefsteak tomatoes. The tomatoes are grown year-round.

The biggest difference between Japanese and American dentists is the cost. In Japan, there is national health insurance whereas in America, it is private and the cost is high. The quality is the same but in Japan, there is more attention to detail and high-tech.

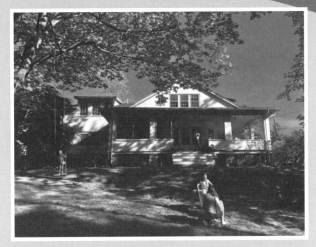
Back home in Boston

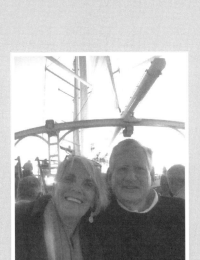
Mom and Dad

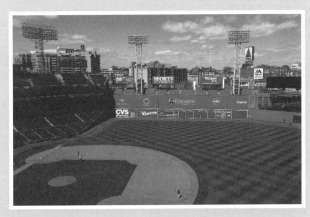
Home of the Boston Red Sox

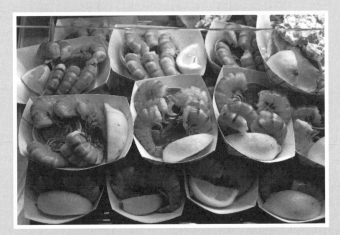
Shrimp cocktail at Quincy Market

The key is to start young and to get as much exposure to English as possible. Daily study, listening to music and watching movies will all help to improve your English.

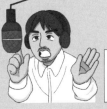

Prosthetics

補綴物

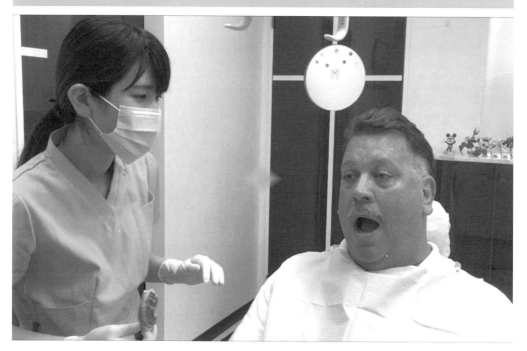

上村先生のワンポイントアドバイス

Our society is increasingly becoming digitalized. In the near future, mixing alginate impression material by hand and swiftly mounting on a tray will become something of the past. However, no matter how technology advances, such basic procedures are important and should be a part of our training.

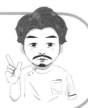

1 Core Terms

次の語を英語の場合は日本語に、日本語の場合は英語に直しなさい。

1. 調節する
2. 金属
3. セラミック
4. 合う (f)

5. 自然な
6. 適合する (m)
7. 置く (p)
8. adhesive

9. esthetic
10. porcelain
11. shade
12. occlusion

13. impression
14. rubbery substance

Brian's Pronunciation Practice
動画の音声に続いてリピートしなさい。

1. adjust	2. metal	3. ceramic	4. fit
5. natural	6. match	7. place	8. adhesive
9. esthetic	10. porcelain	11. shade	12. occlusion
13. impression	14. rubbery substance		

3 Bernie's Pronunciation Tips
患者さんにはクリアな英語を伝える必要があります。
このコーナーでは日本人にとって発音の難しい単語を挙げています。
動画の音声に続いて単語の発音練習をしなさい。

1. berry / very　　2. best / vest　　3. boat / vote　　4. bolt / volt　　5. bet / vet

4 Core Phrases
次の英文を和訳しなさい。

1. Which type of crown do you prefer?

2. Select a color that matches the surrounding teeth.

3. Look at this shade guide.

4. First, I will check the fit.

5. Next, I will examine the bite.

6. Finally, I will attach the crown with adhesive.

7. Use a denture brush to remove food particles.

8. Rinse the denture in lukewarm water.

 Quick Response
動画を見て日本語に対する英訳を瞬時に
口頭で言いなさい。瞬発力が大事です！

Risa's Coffee Break
動画を見ましょう。その後に各器具の名称を英語で書きなさい。

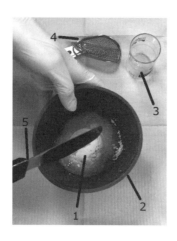

1. アルジネート

2. ラバーボウル

3. 計測カップ

4. トレイ

5. スパチュラ

Workout
以下の症状に該当する診療科を答えなさい。
その後、動画を見てバーニー先生が行くべき診療科を、ブライアン先生と一緒に伝えなさい。

1. My back tooth is growing sideways and needs to be extracted.
2. My cavity seems very deep. It is causing severe pain.
3. My teeth alignment is crowded.
4. My gums are swollen and bleeding.
5. I want artificial teeth that feel like my own.
6. Recently, my bridge doesn't seem to fit right.
7. I need to have my cavity treated.
8. My child has tooth trouble.
9. My grandma's dentures are missing.

Endodontics	Geriatric Dentistry	Implantology
Oral Surgery	Orthodontics	Pediatric Dentistry
Periodontics	Operative Dentistry	Prosthodontics

Dialogs
動画を見て次の各空欄を埋めなさい。

Dialog 1（印象を取ります。）

Dentist: I will (   ) (   ) (   )
　　　　 with this tray filled with rubbery substance.

Patient: Oh, I hate this. It makes me gag.

Dentist: Just try and hold on (   ) (   )
　　　　 (   ) (   ) .

Patient: O.K. I'll try my best.

Dentist: We are finished. You may (   ) (   )
　　　　 your mouth now.

Patient: So, what's next?

Dentist: I am going to put in a (   ) (   ) .
　　　　 We'll be ready to (   ) and (   )
　　　　 the permanent crown a week from now.

Patient: In the (   ) , can I eat as usual?

Dentist: Be careful with (   ) or (   ) food.
　　　　 Also, try to chew (   ) (   ) (   )
　　　　 (   ) .

［注］gag = えづく

Dialog 2（どっちにしようかな？）

Patient: I'm not sure. Which should I choose? (   ) or
　　　　 (   ) ?

Dentist: I think metal will do. It is stronger and I won't have to (   )
　　　　 (   ) too much of the (   )
　　　　 (   ) . On top of that, your (   ) will only
　　　　 cover a metal one.

Patient: Wouldn't it look bad (   ) ?

Dentist: Since the cavity is in the rear, it won't be (   ) ... unless
　　　　 you open your mouth very wide.

Patient: Like when I yawn?

Dentist: But people cover their mouths, don't they?

［注］yawn = あくび

Listening Comprehension
「8」Dialogs の動画をもう一度見て巻末の Answer Sheet にある問題を解きなさい。

10 Test
巻末の Answer Sheet の裏面にあるテストを受けなさい。

Lesson 11
Gum Trouble / Gum Disease
歯肉炎

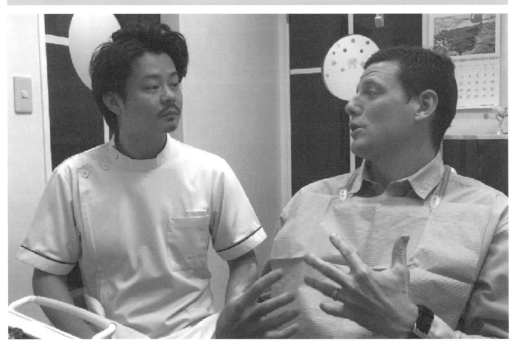

上村先生のワンポイントアドバイス

Along with cavities, periodontal disease can be prevented by daily self care. To assist patients in their self care, many items are available on the market. However, most important is instructions from the dentist on how to correctly conduct the care.

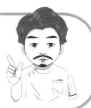

1 Core Terms
次の語を英語の場合は日本語に、日本語の場合は英語に直しなさい。

1. 感染
2. ～で苦しむ
3. 傾向

4. 不適切な
5. 反応
6. gingiva

7. scaling
8. sore（形容詞）
9. calculus

10. periodontal disease
11. recede

2 **Brian's Pronunciation Practice**
動画の音声に続いてリピートしなさい。

1. infection   2. suffer from   3. tendency   4. improper
5. reaction   6. gingiva   7. scaling   8. sore（形容詞）
9. calculus   10. periodontal disease   11. recede

3 **Bernie's Pronunciation Tips**
患者さんにはクリアな英語を伝える必要があります。
このコーナーでは日本人にとって発音の難しい単語を挙げています。
動画の音声に続いて単語の発音練習をしなさい。

1. disease   2. cause   3. incisors   4. resin   5. cleanse

4 **Core Phrases**
次の英文を和訳しなさい。

1. Diabetic patients have a tendency to suffer from periodontal disease.

2. The receding of your gums is caused by improper tooth brushing.

3. My upper front tooth feels loose.

4. Redness of the gums is one of the symptoms of inflammation.

5. Pus is caused by your gums' reaction to bacterial infection.

5 **Quick Response**
動画を見て日本語に対する英訳を瞬時に口頭で言いなさい。
瞬発力が大事です！

Risa's Coffee Break

動画を見て、リサ先生の指示に従いなさい。

その後に写真の器具の名称を英語で書いてみよう。

①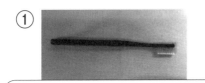

②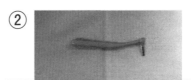

③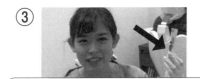

④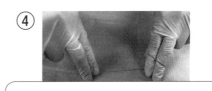

⑤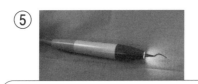

7 **Workout**

hurt は My tooth hurts.「私の歯が痛む」や Where does it hurt?「どこが痛いですか？」というように基本的に動詞の形で使います。

ache はまず My tooth aches.「私の歯が痛む」というように動詞の形で使います。また、toothache「歯痛」や headache「頭痛」といったように痛む箇所の後につなげて名詞の形でも使います。

pain は Where is the pain?「痛いのはどこですか？」や、痛みの種類を表す形容詞を前につけて It is a sharp pain.「鋭い痛みです」といったように主に名詞の形で使います。

 Dialogs

動画を見て次の各空欄を埋めなさい。

Dialog 1（あなたの息ちょっと…。）

A: What did you (　　　　　) (　　　　　) (　　　　　) today?

B: A bowl of clam chowder and some rolls, why?

A: Your breath (　　　　　) (　　　　　) (　　　　　)

onions.

B: Strange. I didn't have any.

A: Maybe (　　　　　) is (　　　　　) (　　　　　)

your gums.

B: Really?

A: Yes, I noticed they look swollen and a bit discolored.

Dialog 2（歯茎の調子が…。）

Patient: My gums have been feeling (　　　　　) (　　　　　)

(　　　　　) lately.

Dentist: Let's see what is going on. Open wide…. There is (　　　　　)

(　　　　　) from your gums.

Patient: Why is that happening?

Dentist: (　　　　　) (　　　　　) (　　　　　)

(　　　　　) infection. I will do some cleaning and disinfect it.

Dialog 3（歯肉トラブルになる前に。）

Dentist: You seem to have (　　　　　) (　　　　　).

Patient: Is it bad?

Dentist: Yes, especially (　　　　　) your lower front teeth. It is causing the

(　　　　　) (　　　　　) your gums.

Patient: How will you treat it?

Dentist: My (　　　　　) will remove the tartar with an

(　　　　　) (　　　　　).

Patient: Will it hurt?

Dentist: Just in case, I will spread some anesthetic around the (　　　　　)

parts.

[注] build up = 堆積

Listening Comprehension

「8」Dialogs の動画をもう一度見て巻末の Answer Sheet にある問題を解きなさい。

10 Test

巻末の Answer Sheet の裏面にあるテストを受けなさい。

Lesson 12
Oral Care Habits
オーラルケア習慣

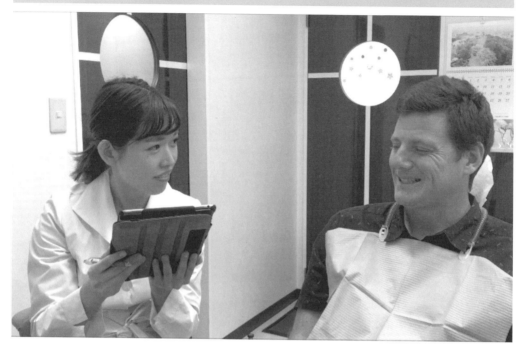

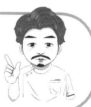

上村先生のワンポイントアドバイス

Correctly understanding the oral care habits of the patient directly influences the outcome of the treatment. Even if what they are doing is incorrect, make sure not to criticize. Rather, encourage the patient and together come up with an "even better" way to improve oral health.

1 Core Terms
次の語を英語の場合は日本語に、日本語の場合は英語に直しなさい。

1. 磨く

2. 歯磨き

3. 食事

4. サプリメント

5. フロス

6. 警告する

7. oral care habits

8. mouthwash

9. medication

10. water pick

2 Brian's Pronunciation Practice
動画の音声に続いてリピートしなさい。

1. brush	2. brushing	3. meal	4. supplement
5. floss	6. warn	7. oral care habits	8. mouthwash
9. medication	10. water pick		

3 Bernie's Pronunciation Tips
患者さんにはクリアな英語を伝える必要があります。
このコーナーでは日本人にとって発音の難しい単語を挙げています。
動画の音声に続いて単語の発音練習をしなさい。

1. supplement　2. sit　3. smooth　4. sore　5. suffer　6. scaling

4 Core Phrases
次の英文を和訳しなさい。

1. When do you brush your teeth?

2. How much time do you spend on each brushing?

3. Do you have any oral care habits besides brushing?

4. Do you smoke?

5. How many hours of sleep do you get on average?

6. Do you eat between meals?

7. Are you receiving any medical treatment now?

8. Are you taking any medication?

5 Quick Response
動画を見て日本語に対する英訳を
瞬時に口頭で言いなさい。瞬発力が大事です！

Risa's Coffee Break
動画を見て、ブライアン先生と一緒に発音しなさい。

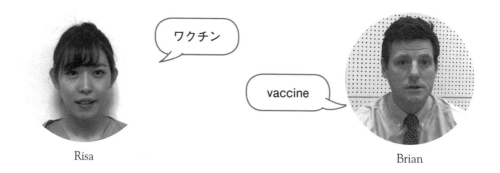

ワクチン

vaccine

Risa

Brian

---

7 Workout
日常生活と歯科医院での英語表現を確認しよう。

▶ ～ is available

日常会話では、
人の場合は、「時間がある」、物の場合は「空きがある」や「入手できる」という
意味になります。
例えば、
Are you available tomorrow?　明日時間ある？
There is a room available for the weekend.　週末の空き部屋が一つあります。
Blue Mountain coffee is available.　ブルーマウンテンコーヒー販売中。

歯科医院では、
予約の曜日や時間の調整をする時に使います。

次の和文を英作しなさい。
１．午後５時からの予約は可能です。

２．明日の午後は歯科衛生士さんがいます。

Dialogs

動画を見て次の各空欄を埋めなさい。

Case 1（お口の手入れについて 1）

Q1: When do you brush your teeth?

A:　(　　　　　　　　　) (　　　　　　　　　) (　　　　　　　　　) .

Q2: How much time do you spend on each brushing?

A:　(　　　　　　　　　) (　　　　　　　　　) (　　　　　　　　　) .

Q3: Do you have any other oral care habits besides brushing?

A:　I (　　　　　　　　　) (　　　　　　　　　) mouthwash.

Q4: Do you smoke?

A:　No, (　　　　　　　　　) (　　　　　　　　　) (　　　　　　　　　) .

Q5: How many hours of sleep do you get on average?

A:　About (　　　　　　　　) (　　　　　　　　) (　　　　　　　　) hours.

Q6: What do you usually drink?

A:　I constantly drink coffee (　　　　　　　　) (　　　　　　　　)

　　(　　　　　　　　) . I also have some wine at dinner time.

Q7: Do you eat between meals?

A:　Sometimes I munch on a bag of potato chips.

Q8: Are you receiving any medical treatment now?

A:　No, I am not.

Q9: Are you taking any medication?

A:　(　　　　　　　　) various supplements, no.

Case 2 (お口の手入れについて 2)

Q1: When do you brush your teeth?

A: In the (　　　　　　) and (　　　　　　) (　　　　　　).

Q2: How much time do you spend on each brushing?

A: (　　　　　) (　　　　　　) (　　　　　)

(　　　　　　) for brushing and then I floss.

Q3: Do you do anything else besides brushing?

A: I use (　　　　　) (　　　　　　) and sometimes a

(　　　　　) (　　　　　).

Q4: Do you smoke?

A: Yes, about (　　　　　) (　　　　　　) (　　　　　)

(　　　　　).

Q5: How many hours of sleep do you get on average?

A: I've been losing sleep because of my busy schedule. I guess about 5 hours

(　　　　　) (　　　　　　) (　　　　　).

Q6: What do you usually drink?

A: I drink (　　　　　) (　　　　　　) (　　　　　)

mineral water. I also like to drink coke.

Q7: Do you eat between meals?

A: No, I don't.

Q8: Are you receiving any medical treatment now?

A: No, but my doctor (　　　　　) (　　　　　)

(　　　　　) my high blood pressure.

Q9: Are you taking any medication?

A: I am (　　　　　) (　　　　　) (　　　　　)

my blood pressure.

Practice
動画（Case1）を見て巻末の Answer Sheet の表面にブライアン先生の質問文を予測して書きなさい。

 Role Playing
巻末の Answer Sheet の裏面を使ってブライアン先生の質問に口頭で答えなさい。尚、答えは自分で用意すること。

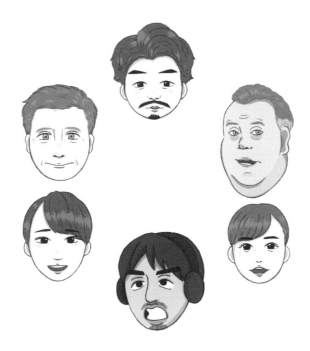

DjD interview program

本日のゲスト ☞ Dr. Naoya Uemura again

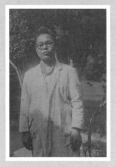
The founder

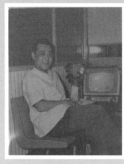
Grandfather

Dr. Uemura, who is a fourth generation dentist, decided to follow his father's footsteps after seeing the satisfied patients showing their appreciation.

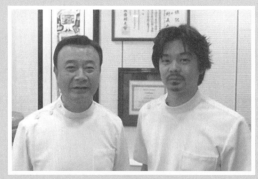
Father and son

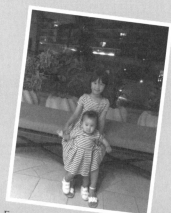
Future dentists?

Elderly patients have a hard time dealing with dentures. Being able to chew again is a joy to these patients.

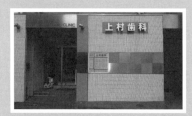

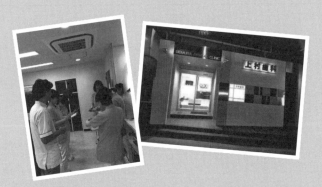

Each morning, Dr. Uemura arrives early and tidies up the clinic. Then he has a staff meeting to go over the treatments and procedures of that day. After lunch break, the afternoon hours start.

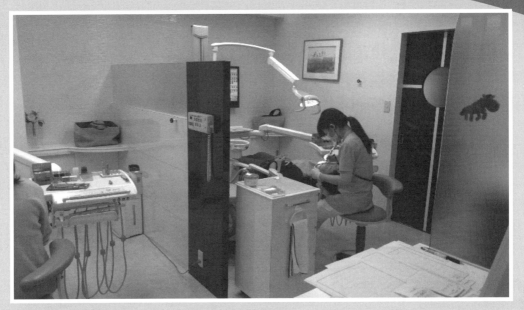

Stamina is important.

When there are not any operations, the day ends with a staff meeting in the early evening.

Treating patients is actual contact with another person. There is much more than what the textbooks say. Patients have different complaints and pains thus it is important for the dentist to listen carefully and communicate.

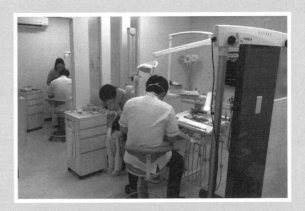

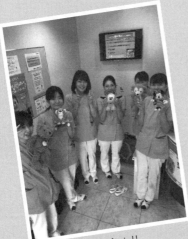

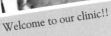

Welcome to our clinic!!

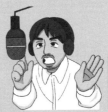

Lesson 13

Giving Advice
患者への指導

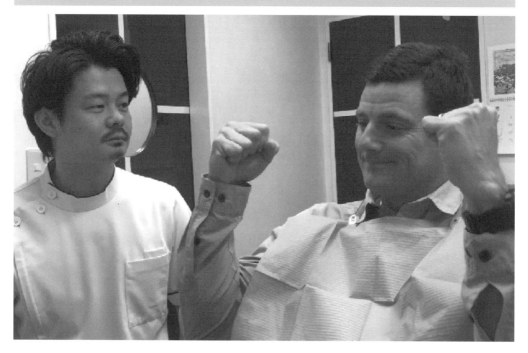

上村先生のワンポイントアドバイス

Following the treatment, the patient is anticipating information about aftercare.
Be sure to provide them with sufficient information such as when they can start
eating or when the pain will go away. Tell them to ask any questions that come
to their minds. Also, encourage them to call whenever they have a problem. This
makes a big difference.

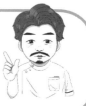

1 Core Terms
次の語を英語の場合は日本語に、日本語の場合は英語に直しなさい。

1. 歯磨き粉	2. 避ける	3. 錠剤	4. 表面
5. 従う	6. 普通の (r)	7. fluoride	8. soft bristles
9. inter-dental brush	10. pain killer	11. antibiotics	12. ointment
13. prescribe	14. prescription	15. just in case	

2   Brian's Pronunciation Practice
動画の音声に続いてリピートしなさい。

1. toothpaste
2. avoid
3. pill
4. surface
5. follow
6. regular
7. fluoride
8. soft bristles
9. inter-dental brush
10. pain killer
11. antibiotics
12. ointment
13. prescribe
14. prescription
15. just in case

3   Bernie's Pronunciation Tips
患者さんにはクリアな英語を伝える必要があります。
このコーナーでは日本人にとって発音の難しい単語を挙げています。
動画の音声に続いて単語の発音練習をしなさい。

（黙字の t） 1. bristles   2. castle   3. hustle   4. wrestle   5. whistle

4   Core Phrases
次の英文を和訳しなさい。

1. Avoid eating hard food.

2. Don't chew on the left side.

3. Don't chew with the treated tooth.

4. Call me if you have any problems.

5. Be sure to follow the prescription.

6. Take one pill three times a day after each meal.

5   Quick Response
動画を見て日本語に対する英訳を瞬時に
口頭で言いなさい。瞬発力が大事です！

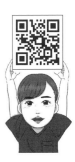

6 Risa's Coffee Break
動画を見て、バーニー先生と一緒に英語で言いなさい。

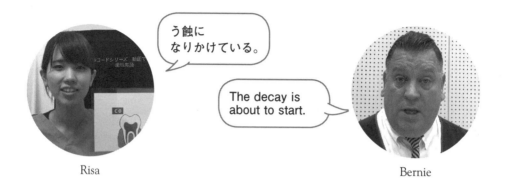

う蝕に
なりかけている。

The decay is
about to start.

Risa

Bernie

---

7 Workout
日常生活と歯科医院での英語表現を確認しよう。

▶ Don't ever... Never...
You may not... Please refrain from...

日常生活では、強い口調で命令する時に使う表現です。

Don't ever come here again.　もう二度と来るな。

Never open that door.　あのドアは絶対に開けるな。

もう少し柔らかい表現になると、

You may not eat or drink in this room.　この部屋での飲食はできません。

Please refrain from eating or drinking in this room.
この部屋での飲食はお控えください。

歯科医院では、

Don't ever use superglue to attach the chipped tooth.

絶対に欠けた歯を瞬間接着材でつけるな。

このように患者に強く注意する時もあるが、

基本的には　"You may not...."（～しないでください）

　　　　　　"Please refrain from...."(～を控えてください) を使う。

次の和文を英作しなさい。

1.一時間は飲食をしないでください。

2.ステインを予防するため喫煙は控えてください。

8 Dialogs
動画を見て次の各空欄を埋めなさい。

Dialog 1 （歯の磨き方について）

Patient:　　How should I brush my teeth correctly?

Dentist:　　Since your gums are (　　　　　　　　), be sure to use a toothbrush

with (　　　　　　) (　　　　　　　).

Patient:　　(　　　　　　) (　　　　　　　　) toothpaste?

Dentist:　　Don't use too much. Regular toothpaste (　　　　　　)

(　　　　　　) (　　　　　　).

Patient:　　Am I brushing too hard?

Dentist:　　(　　　　　) (　　　　　　　) (　　　　　　　)

(　　　　　　　　). Brush softly as if you are raking leaves off the

surface of a rock garden.

Patient:　　Wow! That sounds poetic.

[注] rake = 熊手でかく

Dialog 2 （治療後の注意）

Dentist: I have (　　　　　　　) a temporary filling in the cavity.

Patient: When can I start eating?

Dentist: Be sure to wait (　　　　　　) (　　　　　　) 30 minutes.

Patient: Would it (　　　　　　) (　　　　　　) (　　　　　　)

eat hard food such as almonds?

Dentist: Sure, as long as you (　　　　　　) (　　　　　　)

(　　　　　　) the right side.

Patient: Will it start hurting again?

Dentist: I don't think so, but I have prescribed some (　　　　　　)

(　　　　　　), (　　　　　　), and (　　　　　　) just

in case.

9 Listening Comprehension
動画をもう一度見て巻末の Answer Sheet にある問題を解きなさい。

10 Test
巻末の Answer Sheet の裏面にあるテストを受けなさい。

Lesson 14
Payment and Appointment
支払いと次回の予約

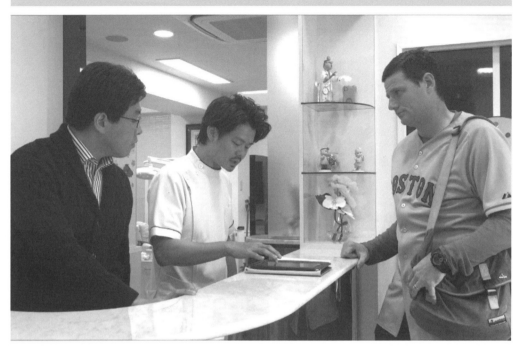

上村先生のワンポイントアドバイス

The management of time is especially important in dental treatment. For instance, when deciding on the next appointment, dentists need to consider the time necessary to prepare prosthesis. Also, if there is too much time in between appointments, the prosthesis may not fit anymore.

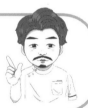

1 Core Terms
次の語を英語の場合は日本語に、日本語の場合は英語に直しなさい。

1. 現金のみ	2. 受けつける	3. クレジットカード	
4. キャンセル	5. 都合のよい	6. より後の	
7. payment	8. bill	9. postpone	10. reception
11. total cost	12. available	13. directions	

2 Brian's Pronunciation Practice
動画の音声に続いてリピートしなさい。

1. cash only
2. accept
3. credit card
4. cancel
5. convenient
6. later
7. payment
8. bill
9. postpone
10. reception
11. total cost
12. available
13. directions

3 Bernie's Pronunciation Tips
患者さんにはクリアな英語を伝える必要があります。
このコーナーでは日本人にとって発音の難しい単語を挙げています。
動画の音声に続いて単語の発音練習をしなさい。

1. ca<u>sh</u>　2. bru<u>sh</u>　3. <u>sh</u>ade　4. poli<u>sh</u>　5. <u>sh</u>arp

4 Core Phrases
次の英文を和訳しなさい。

1. Could you give me directions?

2. Go straight and turn left at the Chinese restaurant.

3. When can you come for the next treatment?

4. What time would be convenient?

5. How about Saturday next week at 5 pm?

6. 5:30 is also available.

5 Quick Response
動画を見て日本語に対する英訳を瞬時に
口頭で言いなさい。瞬発力が大事です！

6 Risa's Coffee Break
動画を見て、バーニー先生と一緒に英語で言いなさい。

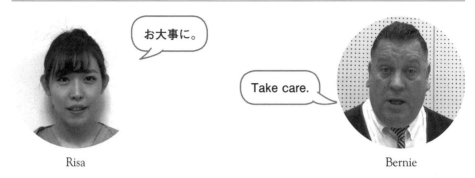

お大事に。

Take care.

Risa

Bernie

7 Workout
日常生活と歯科医院での英語表現を確認しよう。

English

■**抗菌薬　antimicrobial drug**

1回1錠を毎食後に3日間飲んでください。

Take (　　　　　　　) tablet (　　　　　　　) (　　　　　　　)

(　　　　　　　) (　　　　　　　) after each meal.

必ず飲み切ってください。

Be (　　　　　　) (　　　　　　) (　　　　　　) all the medicine.

■**鎮痛剤　pain killer**

痛みが出た場合は1錠ずつ飲んでください。

Take (　　　　　　) tablet (　　　　　　) you have pain.

■**含嗽薬（がんそうやく）　mouthwash**

抜歯したあとの傷口が治るまでの間、1日数回口の中を消毒してください。

(　　　　　　) (　　　　　　) mouthwash (　　　　　　)

(　　　　　　) (　　　　　　) (　　　　　　) until the

extraction site heals.

■**ステロイド　steroids**

口内炎の患部に1日数回塗布してください。

(　　　　　　) (　　　　　　) the canker sores several times a day.

■**抗ヘルペスウイルス薬　anti-herpesvirus drug**

5日間、1日1回食後に服用してください。

Take one tablet a day for five days (　　　　　　) (　　　　　　) .

65

8 Dialogs
動画を見て次の各空欄を埋めなさい。

Dialog 1 （クレジットカードで）

Receptionist: Mr. Parker?

Patient: Yes.

Receptionist: (   ) (   ) (   ) bill.

Patient: Is this covered by my Kokuminhoken, my (   )
               (   ) (   ) ?

Receptionist: Yes it is. You pay (   ) (   ) of the total cost.

Patient: So, how much is it?

Receptionist: It all comes to (   ) (   ) .

Patient: Do you accept credit card?

Receptionist: Yes, we do.

Dialog 2 （次回の予約）

Receptionist: When can you come for the next treatment?

Patient: I can come (   ) (   ) and
               (   ) (   ) .

Receptionist: What time would be convenient?

Patient: (   ) (   ) (   )
               (   ) .

Receptionist: How about Friday next week at 7 pm?

Patient: Do you have anything later than that?

Receptionist: Well, 7:30 (   ) also (   ) .

Patient: O.K. I would like to (   ) (   )
               (   ) at that time.

9 Listening Comprehension
動画をもう一度見て巻末の Answer Sheet にある問題を解きなさい。

10 Test
巻末の Answer Sheet の裏面にあるテストを受けなさい。

Lesson 1: Treatment Procedures

Dialog 1

Q1.   What is the patient's problem?

Q2.   What must he bring to the clinic?

Dialog 2

Q1.   How is the weather?

Q2.   How did the patient find his way to the clinic?

Lesson 1: Treatment Procedures
単語テスト

次の語を英語にしなさい。

1. 開ける

2. 閉じる

3. 噛み合わせる（2単語で）

4. 大きく口を開ける（2単語で）

5. 開けたままにする（2単語で）

6. ゆすぐ

7. 手順

8. 下げる

9. 上げる

10. 治療

Lesson 2: General Terms

Dialog 1

Q1. What did the friend notice about his teeth?

Q2. What seems to be the cause of the problem?

Q3. What does the man like about his dentist?

Dialog 2

Q1. How often does he visit a dental clinic?

Q2. What does this man like about his dentist?

Lesson 2: General Terms
単語テスト

次の語を英語にしなさい。

1. 歯

2. 虫歯

3. 歯科医院（2単語）

4. 歯科医師

5. 歯科医学

6. 脱落

7. 萌出

8. 乳歯（2単語で）

9. 永久歯（2単語で）

10. 着色

Lesson 3: Parts of the Mouth

Dialog 1

Q1.   What kind of emergency is it?

Q2.   What did the patient suggest?

Q3.   Until treatment is available, what precautions should be taken by the patient?

Dialog 2

Q1.   Where is the canker sore?

Q2.   What will the dentist do?

Lesson 3: Parts of the Mouth
単語テスト

次の語を英語にしなさい。

1. 舌

2. （顎）関節

3. 歯肉

4. 歯根

5. 歯冠

6. 犬歯

7. 臼歯

8. 小臼歯

9. 切歯

10. 唾液

Lesson 4: Interview

動画を見て、バーニー先生の質問文を予測して<u>書きなさい</u>。

Case 1

1. Bernie : <u>What seems...?</u>
    Brian : 歯痛

2. Bernie : <u>Is this...?</u>
    Brian : 初めての来院

3. Bernie : <u>Where...?</u>
    Brian : 左下の奥が痛む

4. Bernie : <u>When...?</u>
    Brian : 昨晩から痛む

5. Bernie : <u>What kind...?</u>
    Brian : 鈍い痛み

6. Bernie : <u>Have you ever...?</u>
    Brian : 抜歯の経験あり

7. Bernie : <u>Did you...?</u>
    Brian : 異常なし

Lesson 4: Interview

ブライアン先生の質問文を動画に合わせて<u>言ってみよう</u>。

Case 2

1. Brian : <u>What seems...?</u>
   Bernie : 歯痛

2. Brian : <u>Is this...?</u>
   Bernie : 初めての来院

3. Brian : <u>Where...?</u>
   Bernie : 右上、奥から2番目が痛む

4. Brian : <u>When...?</u>
   Bernie : 先週から痛む

5. Brian : <u>What kind...?</u>
   Bernie : 鋭い痛み

6. Brian : <u>Have you ever...?</u>
   Bernie : 抜歯経験あり

7. Brian : <u>Did you...?</u>
   Bernie : 異常なし

Lesson 5: Interview 2

問診の英語を書きなさい。

1. アレルギーはありますか。
   Do you...?

2. 薬を飲んで副作用は。
   Have you experienced...?

3. 他に気になるところはありますか。
   Is there anything else...?

4. 健康保険の範囲で治しますか。
   Do you have...?

Lesson 5: Interview 2

動画を見て、バーニー先生とブライアン先生の質問文を予測して言いなさい。

Case 1

1. たまごアレルギー

2. 副作用なし

3. 歯茎が腫れている

4. 入っています

Case 2

1. 金属アレルギー

2. 副作用なし

3. 歯がぐらつく

4. 入っています

Lesson 6: Examination

Dialog 1

Q1.   What are the symptoms?

Q2.   When is the appointment?

Dialog 2

Q1.   What is the patient's problem?

Q2.   What is plaque?

Q3.   What would be effective to remove plaque?

Lesson 6: Examination
単語テスト

次の語を英語にしなさい。

1. レントゲン

2. 予約 (a)

3. 細菌

4. 診察

5. 歯列

6. 敏感さ

7. 歯周ポケット（2単語で）

8. 深さ

9. 歯垢

10. 歯間ブラシ（2単語で）

Lesson 7: Diagnosis

Dialog 1

Q1.   What kind of symptoms does the patient have?

Q2.   What did the dentist do before seeing what is wrong?

Q3.   What was the patient's response?

Q4.   What is the diagnosis?

Dialog 2

Q1.   What are the patient's symptoms?

Q2.   What did the dentist do to check?

Q3.   What is the diagnosis?

Lesson 7: Diagnosis
単語テスト

次の語を英語にしなさい。

1. 診断

2. 細菌感染（2 単語で）

3. 口腔乾燥症（2 単語で）

4. 口臭（2 単語で）

5. う蝕

6. 炎症

7. 脱灰

8. 歯周炎

9. 歯肉後退（2 単語で）

10. 膿

Lesson 8: Treatment Procedures 2

Dialog 1

Q1.   What happened to the patient?

Q2.   How will the dentist treat him?

Dialog 2

Q1.   What did the patient feel when he ran his tongue over the filling?

Q2.   What did the dentist do to solve the problem?

Q3.   What did the patient say about the adjustment?

Lesson 8: Treatment Procedures 2
単語テスト

次の語を英語にしなさい。

1. 前後（3単語で）

2. 左右

3. 荒い

4. うがい

5. 噛みしめる

6. ギリギリさせる

7. 凹凸や角（3単語で）

8. コンポジットレジン（2単語で）

9. 接着する

10. 磨く

Lesson 9: Treating Cavities

Dialog 1

Q1.   What symptoms is the patient complaining about?

Q2.   What is the result of the x-ray?

Q3.   What kind of treatment did the dentist suggest?

Dialog 2

Q1.   Why does the patient need root canal treatment?

Q2.   What is the procedure of the treatment?

Q3.   How does the dentist explain about the pain of the treatment?

Lesson 9: Treating Cavities
単語テスト

次の語を英語にしなさい。

1. 深い

2. 削る

3. 消毒する

4. 充填する

5. カリエス

6. 仮留め（2単語で）

7. 充填（2単語で）

8. 根管（2単語で）

9. 破折

10. 洗浄する

Lesson 10: Prosthetics

Dialog 1

Q1.   Why is the patient reluctant to take an impression?

Q2.   What kind of treatment will the dentist do for that day?

Q3.   What should the patient be careful of?

Dialog 2

Q1.   What are the three reasons why the dentist recommends a metal crown?

Q2.   What is the patient worried about concerning metal crowns?

Q3.   Why does the dentist think the patient's worry is not a problem?

Lesson 10: Prosthetics
単語テスト

次の語を英語にしなさい。

1. 調節する

2. 金属

3. セラミック

4. 自然な

5. 置く (p)

6. 審美的な

7. 陶材

8. 色調

9. 咬合 (o)

10. 印象

Lesson 11: Gum Trouble / Gum Disease

Dialog 1

Q1.   What is wrong with the man's breath?

Q2.   How do his gums appear?

Dialog 2

Q1.   What is the patient's complaint?

Q2.   What did the dentist see inside the patient's mouth?

Q3.   How will the condition be treated?

Dialog 3

Q1.   What is the patient's problem?

Q2.   What kind of treatment will be conducted?

Q3.   What precaution will be taken?

Lesson 11: Gum Trouble / Gum Disease
単語テスト

次の語を英語にしなさい。

1. 感染

2. ～で苦しむ（2単語で）

3. 傾向

4. 不適切な

5. 反応

6. 歯肉

7. スケーリング

8. 痛い (s)

9. 歯石 (c)

10. 歯周病（2単語で）

Lesson 12: Oral Care Habits

問診の英語を書きなさい。

Case 1

Q1:   When....

I brush my teeth after each meal.

Q2:   How much time....

I spend about 5 minutes on each brushing.

Q3:   Do you have any.... (歯磨き以外の口腔衛生習慣)

I use mouthwash.

Q4:   Do you.... (喫煙)

No, I don't.

Q5:   How many hours.... (平均睡眠時間)

I would say about 6 hours.

Q6:   What.... (よく飲むもの)

I am a serious coffee drinker!

Q7:   Do you.... (間食)

I love jellybeans.

Q8:   Are you receiving.... (他の治療)

I am seeing my doctor for diabetes.

Q9:   Are you taking.... (投薬)

Yes, what my doctor prescribes.

Lesson 12: Oral Care Habits

お口のお手入れに関する質問に対して、動画（Case2）に合わせて自分で答えを用意して言ってみなさい。

Case 2

Q1:　When do you brush your teeth?

Q2:　How much time do you spend on each brushing?

Q3:　Do you have any other oral care habits besides brushing?

Q4:　Do you smoke?

Q5:　How many hours of sleep do you get on average?

Q6:　What do you usually drink?

Q7:　Do you eat between meals?

Q8:　Are you receiving any medical treatment now?

Q9:　Are you taking any medication?

Lesson 13: Giving Advice

Dialog 1

Q1.   What kind of toothbrush is recommended?

Q2.   What about toothpaste?

Q3.   How should the patient brush?

Dialog 2

Q1.   What precautions should the patient take?

Q2.   What did the dentist prescribe, just in case?

Lesson 13: Giving Advice
単語テスト

次の語を英語にしなさい。

1. 歯磨き粉

2. 避ける

3. 表面

4. フッ化物

5. 柔らかい毛先（2単語で）

6. 痛み止め（2単語で）

7. 抗生剤

8. 軟膏

9. 処方する

10. 処方箋

Lesson 14: Payment and Appointment

Dialog 1

Q1.   What kind of insurance does the patient have?

Q2.   What percentage must he pay?

Q3.   How will he pay?

Dialog 2

Q1.   When will the next appointment be?

Lesson 14: Payment and Appointment
単語テスト

次の語を英語にしなさい。

1. 現金のみ（2単語で）

2. 受け付ける (a)

3. 都合のよい (c)

4. 支払い

5. 請求書

6. 延期

7. 受付

8. 合計金額（2単語で）

9. 利用可能 (a)

10. 道順

歯科医学英語ワークブック　第2版
QRコードで動画が見られる!

2015年5月15日　第1版 第1刷
2018年3月20日　第1版 第2刷
2020年3月15日　第2版 第1刷 ©

著　者	藤田淳一	FUJITA, Junichi
	岡 隼人	OKA, Hayato
発行者	宇山閑文	
発行所	株式会社金芳堂	

〒606-8425 京都市左京区鹿ケ谷西寺ノ前町34番地
振替　01030-1-15605
電話　075-751-1111 （代）
https://www.kinpodo-pub.co.jp/

組　版	HON DESIGN
印刷・製本	モリモト印刷株式会社

落丁・乱丁本は直接小社へお送りください. お取替え致します.

Printed in Japan
ISBN978-4-7653-1811-2